The A–Z of
School Health

The A–Z of
School Health

Adrian Brooke

and Steve Welton

David Fulton Publishers
London

David Fulton Publishers Ltd
The Chiswick Centre, 414 Chiswick High Road, London W4 5TF

www.fultonpublishers.co.uk

David Fulton Publishers is a division of Granada Learning, part of the Granada Media group

First published 2003
10 9 8 7 6 5 4 3 2 1

Copyright © 2003 Adrian Brooke and Steve Welton

British Library Cataloguing in Publication Data
A catalogue record for this book is available from the British Library.

ISBN 1 85346 830 4

Typeset by Book Production Services, London
Printed and bound in Scotland by Scotprint, Haddington

Contents

Introduction

This book aims to provide basic information about medical conditions that affect learning. It describes symptoms and signs, and outlines current key concepts in educational medicine. It also gives information on conditions and provides signposts to aid the recognition and delineation of the associated problems that might affect learning. Uniquely, the book also provides educational approaches taken to accommodate children with the conditions and problems listed. As many children with special educational needs might not have a specific diagnosis, the book takes a problem-orientated approach where appropriate. The book's combined medical and educational perspectives are designed to provide those working with children with healthcare needs with easily accessible information.

Why this book?

There are many reasons why information and a basic knowledge on the health of children are becoming more important.

- There are an increasing number of medical conditions that impact upon the education of children and young people.
- With improvements in medical knowledge and technology, more children with complex health needs are attending mainstream schools.
- By the same token, children who previously might have not survived now live through childhood and beyond, and therefore need suitable education to enhance their life skills and potential.
- The continuing emphasis on integration and inclusion in education enshrined in recent legislation will mean that more children with more complex healthcare needs are likely to receive their education in a mainstream setting.
- With the greater emphasis on academic success as a key to achieving in later life, doctors are being asked more often by parents to see if there are medical or other remediable causes for their child's difficulties at school.
- Conditions previously known about in only a few children are now being increasingly recognised and in turn have led to the new morbidities to which both medicine and education struggle to adapt.

- Media interest and publicity, combined with increased parental knowledge and expectation, have led to an increased demand for focused and expert assessment of conditions that impact upon the educational experiences of the child. Much of the assessment of children with educational problems of whatever cause requires timely and accurate information from teachers and others involved in a child's learning.
- In order to enhance communication with, and understanding of, healthcare professionals, a basic understanding of the vocabulary, concepts and limitations of clinical method as applied to educational medicine are required.

This A–Z allows rapid reference to conditions commonly encountered in school-aged children and also to more rare diseases, focusing particularly on the impact of the condition on the child's access to the curriculum. It also offers practical advice on some educational approaches that are used to support children's learning. Links to further information including websites follow many entries.

Readership

The book will be essential reading for teachers, head teachers, SENCOs, educational managers, assessment officers, and any person involved with meeting the special educational needs of children. It will be a useful reference work for other associated professionals and an invaluable resource for doctors, school nurses and therapists working with children in school, and finally parents themselves.

It is hoped that most SENCOs will want a copy as a handy reference guide. A book like this is timely as the government pushes for further integration and inclusion in mainstream educational settings, as public knowledge of medical conditions increases and as expectations for educational achievement are increased.

The structure of the book

The book is intended to be used for specific reference when seeking information about children and young people in educational settings. Sources of further information are provided at the end of most entries.

The book is largely an alphabetically organised list of medical conditions; during the process of compiling entries, three aspects frequently recurred and have therefore been given separate attention in the chapters on the language of medicine and education, legislation and working with other agencies.

How to use the book

When seeking information on a condition, go to the A–Z section and find the entry; alternatively look in the index for the page number. Individual entries are generally in the following order:

- medical information
- implications for the child

- considerations for education and finally useful links.

Note that all medical information used in schools needs to be checked and agreed by the school's medical advisers. There is no better information than the highly individual information about the child or young person that can be provided by parents and by well-kept records.

Further information or no information

For further information there are addresses and websites at the end of each entry. If there is not an entry for a condition, then further information should be available from the school doctor or other healthcare professional. As time goes on, more information is becoming available via the Internet; although it is important to be aware that the Internet is an unregulated medium and therefore the quality and reliability of information obtained cannot be guaranteed. The Internet is a vast source of medical information much of which is not endorsed. For good dependable information, use sites that subscribe to the guidelines of *Health on the Net* – these can be found on the HON site (www.hon.ch). Further information containing guidance on checking quality of health websites can be

found at www.hiquality.org.uk. In the UK a very useful resource for information is the CAF (Contact a Family) directory www.cafamily.co.uk.

The book deliberately does not contain information about many temporary conditions or illnesses that require children and young people to be absent from school.

Further contributions

In putting this handbook together we have had to make decisions about what to include. It has been difficult in some circumstances to decide what potential readers might need to know and what information would be most useful. We would be most interested to hear of suggestions for additions and amendments to make future editions more useful. Please contact us via the publishers.

Disclaimer

While every effort has been made to ensure the accuracy of the contents, we cannot be held responsible for any errors or omissions. Any medical information is provided for educational/information purposes only. Readers should obtain further information and advice from a medical practitioner as appropriate.

Acknowledgements

The authors would like to thank the following people who read sections/chapters and made helpful suggestions: Mike Silverman, Professor of Child Health at the University of Leicester; Dawn Adams, Teacher of the Visually Impaired, Leicestershire; Colin Bowpitt, SENCO, Shenton Primary School, Leicester; Tony Smith, Head Teacher, Dorothy Goodman School, Hinckley; the children, their families and valued colleagues with whom we have worked for many years in Leicester and Leicestershire.

Finally, our families deserve special thanks – this time should have been yours.

1 The language of medicine and education

The language of medicine

It is estimated that doctors learn more new words in their undergraduate education than foreign language students. Medicine and medical practice has developed over thousands of years and the language has, consequently, grown with it. Many medical terms are derived from Latin or Greek, although other conditions take their name from still different languages. The complexity of human health and disease requires an enormous vocabulary to describe it accurately, adequately and reliably to other health professionals. Many medical terms have found their way into the general language and therefore become used in a different way. An example would be 'chronic'. Doctors use this word to describe conditions that last a long time, whereas others might use it to describe how severe a condition was. Herein lies a potential communication problem between doctors and their patients.

Patients sometimes describe symptoms using medical words, assuming that they are helping the doctor by doing so. However, this might in fact serve only to confuse the issue if the doctor has a different understanding to the medical word or phrase that the patient uses. For example, a child may be described by the parent as being 'hyperactive', or even just 'hyper'. To the doctor the term 'hyperactive' means a high level of motor activity that is defined by many behavioural, environmental and developmental criteria. It is therefore easy to see that the parent's description of the child might not echo the assessment of the doctor, even though they may both be using the same medical words.

Whilst the highly developed language of medicine is useful for communication between professionals, it can be used to exclude those who do not understand the language fully. In these circumstances the language acts as a barrier to effective communication and care rather than an aid.

It is in an attempt to explain some of the medical terminology and medical conditions that this book has been written. It is hoped that by demystifying some of the (sometimes arcane) language of medicine, communication between educationalists and health professionals can be improved to the benefit of the children concerned.

The language of education

Education, like many professions, has evolved its own language including its specialised terms and phrases. It comprises jargon, which is useful to teachers and others in education, but can be less than helpful to outsiders. Children, parents, carers and colleagues do need to communicate with teachers and others working in the field of education. At times the educational jargon used by some teachers is not helpful and the technical terms used by some specialist educationalists can be impenetrable.

Teachers and educationalists use a language that blossomed in the twentieth century and is littered with the words and ideas that come from within the various influences that have come to bear on education. Many teachers will use words borrowed from the disciplines of sociology, psychology and, more rarely, philosophy. Added to this are words derived from the 'speak' of the most recent 'gurus' of business and commerce, as successive governments have sought to apply the tools and methodologies of the market place. It is not unusual therefore to hear teachers using words associated with business management, accountancy, architecture and the military, for example, to describe things in schools. Teachers together might be quite comfortable exchanging views on 'opportunities for open learning in a child-centred setting' or, 'interactive strategies', or the importance of the school's 'resource deployment capability'. This use of jargon between the initiated is possibly quite useful for teachers, and confirms belonging to the group with an awareness of current educational issues. However, when this kind of belonging means denying access to others, it is unlikely to be of benefit to those for whom the language has been developed.

Teachers who use jargon unnecessarily are not helping communication or their relationships with non-educationalists. It is very important for all teachers and others involved in education to use plain English and to take pains to be good at simple communication both in and out the classroom.

A list of some words and terms that have caused confusion or required explanation

AEN Additional Educational Needs

Appropriate education When a child is taught in the way and at the rate that the child learns best

Assessment A systematic way of finding out what a child can and cannot do

Attention span The length of time that someone concentrates on a task without being distracted or losing interest

Audit Stocktaking or listing provision or things in a financial sense

Auditory association The ability to understand, comprehend and use spoken language appropriately

Auditory discrimination The learned ability to recognise and understand differences in sounds. This is to do with interpreting what is heard rather than what has actually been heard

Auditory figure-ground Ability to pay attention to one sound and shut out unimportant background noise

Auditory memory The ability to remember and recall what has been said. *Short-term auditory memory* is the ability to recall what has been said immediately before; *long-term auditory memory* is the ability to recall what has been said more than a minute previously. *Sequential auditory memory* is the recall of a number of pieces of information in the correct order

Auditory perception The ability to understand that which is heard

Baseline assessment The assessment of a child's aptitude and ability on starting school

Benchmarking A standard or a point of reference against which pupil achievement can be assessed

Body awareness Being aware of where the body is in relation to space, movement and other objects

Broad and balanced curriculum All subjects need to be taught: English, Mathematics, Science and Information Technology are most important and should take up a large part of a pupil's time, but other subjects must have sufficient time spent on them

CAN (Complex Additional Needs) The description of pupils and students with sensory impairment and other serious conditions

Carer The person with parental responsibility

Casework officer An officer of the Local Education Authority who liaises with the parents and others during the process relating to Statutory Assessment and the making of a Statement of Special Educational Needs

Circle time A technique for raising pupils' self-esteem in school

The Code of Practice There are various codes of practice. In the context of special education, this includes the detailed procedures for the assessment and recording of special educational needs

Cognition The mental process or act whereby knowledge is acquired

Cognitive skills Skills related to knowing and understanding such as perception, intuition and thinking

Cohort A group of pupils

Communication disorder A disorder that prevents communication or understanding of communication

Conceptualisation The ability to see a number of linked items and form an idea about them, such as recognising attributes of colour, shape or size

Connexions Connexions brings together a full range of youth support services so that young people aged 13–19 years can overcome barriers to their education, training and employment opportunities. Every young person will have access to a 'Personal Adviser' to assist them in making a smooth transition to adult services

Cross dominance Where the preferred eye, hand, foot or ear is on different sides of the body; for example, a child might write with the right hand but play tennis with the left

Decoding The ability to obtain meaning from written words, letters, numbers or symbols

DfES Department for Education and Skills

Differentiation Work presented at a variety of levels to suit pupils' different levels of ability in group or class settings

Discrimination The ability to notice the differences and similarities between various things

EBD Emotional and Behavioural Difficulties

EDP Education Development Plan A requirement by the government for local plans for educational development

Encoding The ability to find the right words, numbers or symbols and use them to form ideas or to produce them in writing or speech

EP Educational Psychologist

EWO Education Welfare Officer

Expressive language The ability to communicate appropriately using body language, speech or writing

FE Further Education

FEFC Further Education Funding Council replaced by the **Learning Skills Council**

Fine motor The use of small muscles for a detailed series of actions such as writing or doing up shoelaces

Gross motor The use of large muscles for actions that involve larger parts of the body such as walking and running

Hand–eye coordination The ability to use both eyes and hands together to perform a task such as writing, drawing, cutting paper doing up shoe laces

HE Higher Education

HI Hearing Impairment

ICT Information and Communication Technology

IEP Individual Education Plan Short-term learning targets set down for a child with special educational needs; this is usually put together by the SEN Coordinator, teachers, parents and pupils

Inclusion The process of ensuring that defined groups within school are included in all that happens. Inclusion is also used to describe educating all children, including those with special educational needs, in mainstream (local) schools, and to describe the means by which young people and adults with disabilities and/or learning difficulties are included in mainstream society

Integration A term used previously to describe inclusion

Joined-up thinking Departments working together – particularly education, social services and health

Laterality The awareness and knowledge that two sides of the body are different and can be moved individually or together in different actions. A common cause of underachievement at school is inadequately developed laterality where children are slow to learn their left and right sides

LEA Local Education Authority

LSC Learning Skills Council Regional councils to replace the Further Education Funding Council and the Training and Enterprise Councils and deal with all issues relating to funding and training post-16-year-old children

Mixed laterality Where a person changes from right to left side during or for certain activities rather than using a preferred side

MLD Moderate Learning Difficulties

Mnemonic device A way of helping the memory by linking images, words, rhymes or ideas

Modality The sense through which information is acquired such as hearing, smell, sight, touch and taste

Motor To do with movement of parts of the body

Motor coordination The ability to use muscle groups together to carry out movements

Motor planning The mental planning required before the body is able to do a series of movements or actions

Multi-agency More than one agency, such as Education, Health and Family, and Community Services

Multidisciplinary Involving professionals from a range of departments or disciplines usually Education, Social Services, and Health

Multisensory Involving some or all of the senses

MSI/MNSI Multi Sensory Impairment or MultiNeeds Sensory Impairment

Norm referenced tests Performance tests that can be used to make comparisons between pupils of the same age. IQ tests and most achievement tests are norm referenced

Oral language Spoken language

Peripheral vision The ability to see from the edge of the eyes to the sides while looking directly at something in front

PMLD Profound and Multiple Learning Difficulties

Portage A planned approach to home based preschool education for children with special educational needs

Primitive reflexes The reflexes that newly born babies have designed to enable them to survive and develop in the early weeks and months of life. They are usually present for a limited time and help the baby through early development. They usually disappear or become 'inhibited', allowing more complex neural structures to develop. If these primitive reflexes continue to be present, they are termed 'aberrant', indicating a weakness or immaturity within the central nervous system

Proprioception Knowing where the position of body or parts of the body are in space and knowing where they are when they are moved

Receptive language Understanding what others say

Reflex An instinctive response to sensory stimulation such as blinking or widening of the pupils of the eye

SALT Speech And Language Therapist

Semantics The meaning of spoken or written language

SEN Special Educational Needs

SENCO Special Educational Needs Coordinator The member of staff who has responsibility for coordinating special educational needs provision within the school

Sensorimotor The relationship between movement and the sensations or signals sent to the brain as a result

SI Sensory Impairment

SLD Severe Learning Difficulties

Spatial orientation The awareness of space around a person relative to position, distance and direction

Standardised test Performance tests that can be used to make comparisons between pupils of the same age. IQ tests and most achievement tests are standardised

Tactile defensiveness The defensive reaction to unexpected stimuli

Task analysis The ability to break a task down into its processes and parts

Tracking The ability to follow a moving object such as a light beam or a line of writing with the eyes

Transition plan The action plan for transition to adult life following the review of a young person's special educational needs at the age of 14 years

Transposition Where letters or numbers are confused

TTA Teacher Training Agency

Vestibular system or sense Knowing the head's position and movement in space, which affects posture and balance

Visual discrimination The ability to notice and understand differences in what is seen

Visual motor Ability to translate information received visually into a motor response, such as copying from a book or blackboard

2 Recent legislation

Definitions of special needs

Recent legislation has defined special needs, special educational needs and disability. The *Special Educational Needs and Disability Act 2001* and the *SEN Code of Practice* are the most recent sources of definitions; however, earlier Acts provide slightly different understandings as follows.

Education Act 1996, Section 312

Children have special educational needs if they have a learning difficulty which calls for special educational provision to be made for them.
Children have a learning difficulty if they:
(a) have significantly greater difficulty in learning than the majority of children of the same age; or
(b) have a disability which prevents or hinders the child from making use of educational facilities of a kind generally provided for children of the same age in schools within the area of the local education authority; or
(c) are under compulsory school age and fall within the definition at (a) or (b) above or would do so if special educational provision was not made for them.
Children must not be regarded as having a learn-ing difficulty solely because the language or form of language of their home is different from the language in which they will be taught.

Special educational provision means:

for children of two or over, educational provision which is additional to, or otherwise different from, the educational provision made generally for children of their age in schools maintained by the LEA, other than special schools, in the area for children under two, educational provision of any kind

Children Act 1989, Section 17(11)

A child is disabled if he is blind, deaf or dumb or suffers from a mental disorder of any kind or is substantially and permanently handicapped by illness, injury or congenital deformity or such other disability as may be prescribed

Disability Discrimination Act 1995, Section 1(1)

A person has a disability for the purposes of this Act if he has a physical or mental impairment which has a substantial and long-term adverse effect on his abil-ity to carry out normal day-to-day activities.

It should be noted that children may fall within one or more of these definitions. Children with a disability will have special educational needs if they have any difficulty accessing education and if they need any special educational provision made for them.

Special Educational Needs and Disability Act 2001

The *Special Educational Needs and Disability Act* will begin to come into effect from 1 September 2002. The Act removes the previous exemption of education from the *Disability Discrimination Act (1995)*, ensuring that discrimination against disabled students is unlawful. Institutions will incur additional responsibilities in 2003, with the final sections of legislation coming into effect in 2005.

This legislation is very much part of the government's commitment to inclusion and strengthens the duty to provide a mainstream place for pupils with SEN where this is what parents wish and is compatible with 'efficient education of other children'.

The Act seeks to prevent discrimination against disabled people regarding their 'access to education' in the widest sense of 'access'. The Act very clearly underpins the SEN Code of Practice 2002.

The key message is to make it unlawful to 'discriminate, without justification, against disabled pupils in all aspects of school life'. Additionally schools might not treat disabled pupils less favourably and must make reasonable adjustments to avoid putting disabled pupils at a substantial disadvantage. The Act indicates that cases of discrimination will not be made against individuals within the school but against the 'responsible body', e.g. governing body or equivalent.

The duty to make reasonable adjustments is a duty to disabled people generally, not just to particular individuals. The 'anticipatory' aspect of this duty means that institutions need to consider what sort of adjustments might be necessary for disabled people in the future and, where appropriate, make these adjustments in advance. It will not be enough to wait until a disabled student requests adjustment(s).

The Act requires LEAs to draw up 'accessibility strategies' and schools to draw up 'accessibility plans' to improve access to education at schools over time. Access includes improvements to curricular access, education and services through attention to physical matters, and to information through appropriate formatting of access information.

The Act covers a range of duties on schools, colleges and LEAs. Comprehensive local information and copies of the Act will be available from schools, libraries, Local Education Authorities, the Department for Education and Skills, or from the Internet.

Key documents for the Special Educational Needs and Disability Act 2001

Special Educational Needs and Disability Act 2001
Download address: www.hmso.gov.uk/acts/acts2001/20010010.htm
Inclusive Schooling – Children with Special Educational Needs

The document provides practical guidance on the new statutory framework for inclusion.

Download address: www.dfes.gov.uk/sen/viewDocument.cfm?dID=237

The SEN Code of Practice 2002

The *SEN Code of Practice* was recently updated following a lengthy consultation process with schools, Education Authorities, parents, and a wide variety of agencies and voluntary bodies. It places a new emphasis on preventative work to ensure that children's special educational needs are identified as quickly as possible and that early action is taken to meet those needs.

The principles of the *SEN Code of Practice* are that:

- All children with SEN should have their needs met.
- Children's needs will normally be met in mainstream schools or early education settings.
- The views of children should be sought and taken into account.
- Parents have a vital role to play in supporting their child's education.
- Children with SEN should be offered full access to a broad, balanced and relevant education, including an appropriate curriculum for the foundation stage and the National Curriculum.

Local Education Authorities need to ensure that:
- The culture, practice, management and deployment of resources are designed to ensure all children's needs are met.
- Schools and settings work with them to ensure that all children's SEN are identified early.

- Schools and settings join them to develop best practice.
- Those responsible for SEN provision take into account the views and wishes of the child.
- Professionals and parents work in partnership.
- Professionals take account of parents' views.
- Provision and progress is monitored and reviewed regularly.
- There is cooperation between all agencies.
- Assessments are made within the prescribed time limits.
- Statements are clear and detailed, specify monitoring arrangements and are reviewed annually.

The revised *Code of Practice* sets out a graduated approach of intervention for children with SEN. **School Action** is in many ways the existing good classroom practice of children having their needs met through differentiation of the curriculum. Where children are not making progress, then teachers should consult more widely with other professionals seeking advice and support. This is known as **School Action Plus**. Where children are still not making progress, then the school or parents should ask the LEA to carry out a statutory assessment. Should the LEA agree, then an assessment will take place within six weeks. The assessment may result in a statement describing the needs and the provision that must be made to meet those needs. If the LEA decides that a statement is not needed, then a child can continue to receive additional help at School Action Plus.

All teachers are teachers of children with special educational needs and will join in identifying children's needs and tailoring teaching approaches to meet those needs.

It should not be assumed that children who are making slower progress must necessarily have special educational needs. All children will need carefully differentiated learning opportunities to help them progress, with regular and frequent careful monitoring of their progress. There should not be an assumption that all children will progress at the same rate. A judgement has to be made in each case as to what it is reasonable to expect that particular child to achieve. Children making slow progress or having particular difficulties in one area might be given extra help, different lessons, different support, help or activities in class to help them to succeed. This differentiation is *not* SEN provision. Teachers' planning should be flexible in order to recognise the needs of all children as individuals and to ensure progression, relevance and differentiation.

Individual Education Plans should have three or four targets, appropriate strategies and a record of the outcomes. The targets should usually relate to the key areas of communication, literacy, mathematics, behaviour and social skills – the strategies will sometimes be cross-curricular and sometimes subject specific. They are meant to be a teaching and planning tool. Where schools have a policy of individual planning and recording for all pupils, then the child with SEN may not need a separate IEP at all. In those schools, perhaps, the interventions for children with SEN will be recorded as part of the class lesson plans, along with a record of the child's progress and the outcomes of the intervention – in the same way as for all the other children. For example, a physically disabled pupil, able to fully access the curriculum and attending a school that is fully accessible, will not need an IEP, but will need progress recorded on an individual basis like all other pupils.

Partnership with parents plays a key role in promoting a culture of cooperation between parents, schools, LEAs and others. Parents hold key information and have a critical role to play in their children's education. They know their child best and have unique strengths, knowledge and experience to contribute to the shared view of a child's needs and the best ways of supporting them. The practice of seeking and taking account of the views of children and young people with SEN is emphasised strongly.

LEAs have strategic roles for SEN and must provide easily accessible information to promote effective monitoring of SEN provision. They should encourage consultation and cooperation with settings, schools and a wide range of other partners including health, social services, and the voluntary sector in developing policies and plans. LEAs need to work with schools to evaluate the effectiveness of their school funding arrangements in supporting and raising the achievement of children with SEN and in developing their policies and provision.

Effective inter-agency working is necessary for children with SEN. The *Code of Practice* makes clear that services must work together to:

- make early identification
- work closely with the child and parents

- provide focused intervention
- disseminate effective approaches and techniques
- plan for the future.

It is beyond the scope of this book to outline in detail the *SEN Code of Practice* and all its related advice. Further information will be available from schools, libraries, Local Education Authorities, the Department for Education and Skills or from the Internet.

Key documents for the SEN Code of Practice 2002

The SEN Code of Practice
The *SEN Code of Practice* provides practical advice to Local Education Authorities, maintained schools, early education settings and others on carrying out their statutory duties to identify, assess and make provision for children's special educational needs.

Download address: www.dfes.gov.uk/sen/index.cfm

The SEN Toolkit 2001
The *SEN Toolkit*, mainly for schools and LEAs, contains practical advice on how to implement the Code. It should be read in conjunction with the Code. Each section of the Toolkit has a number of pages designed to be copied and used as slides for training purposes.

Download address: www.dfes.gov.uk/sen/viewDocument.cfm?dID=263

SEN – A guide for parents and carers
This sets out the main points of the Code of Practice, explains procedures and tells parents their rights. Copies will be available from schools, libraries, Local Education Authorities, the Department for Education and Skills or from the Internet.

Download address: www.dfes.gov.uk/sen/news/viewArticle.cfm?aID=24

Access to Education for Children and Young People with Medical Needs
This sets out minimum national standards for the education of children who are unable to attend school because of illness or injury.

Download address: www.dfes.gov.uk/sen/viewDocument.cfm?dID=257

Key contact information for the *SEN Code of Practice 2002*
Department for Education and Skills
Tel: 08700 012345
Public Enquiries: 0870 000 2288
Publications: 0845 602 2260

LONDON
Department for Education and Skills
Sanctuary Buildings
Great Smith Street
London SW1P 3BT

Department for Education and Skills
Caxton House
Tothill Street
London SW1H 9FN

SHEFFIELD
Department for Education and Skills
Moorfoot
Sheffield S1 4PQ

DARLINGTON
Department for Education and Skills

Mowden Hall
Staindrop Road
Darlington DL3 9BG

RUNCORN
Department for Education and Skills
Castle View House
East Lane
Runcorn WA7 2DN

3 Working with other agencies

By its very nature working with children with healthcare conditions will mean working with a wide range of other workers coming from many disciplines, agencies and professions. In nearly every entry in this handbook there is a reference to interdisciplinary working. Good and well-planned work with others contributes greatly to the positive experience that education needs to be.

Hospital schools

Many children and young people with medical conditions will at some time have their educational needs met through their local hospital school or service. This service provides the necessary tuition for the children admitted to the hospital who are well enough to study, so that when they are well they will encounter less difficulty in resuming their schooling.

Pupils attend hospital schools by arrangement with the doctors in charge of the hospital wards. Those who are less mobile receive individual bedside tuition. Pupils have their lessons in discrete classrooms or in groups in the wards or at home. Some hospital education services provide for pregnant schoolgirls and for patients with psychiatric disorders.

Staff in hospital schools are highly skilled in flexible working; they work across all ages and abilities and need to be familiar with different examination systems. Their work is dependant on effective communication with a patient's school, parents and all others that may be involved.

Interdisciplinary working

School staff meeting the special educational needs of children with medical conditions will need to meet with parents and with professionals from other disciplines. High quality special educational provision for pupils with complex needs is generally characterised by effective interdisciplinary working. The constitution of a multidisciplinary team will depend on the special needs of the child.

The child and parents can be in a situation where they are moved from one profession or service to another with great regularity, having to provide the same information a number of times. Good *Interdisciplinary working* can reduce the numbers of visits for children and parents as well as the need to repeat information. The benefits for the child and those working closely with the child are great, and it is therefore worth planning multidisciplinary meetings with parents.

Getting agencies to work together effectively is very difficult to achieve. A family can have as many as ten to fifteen professionals involved in their child at any one time. The differences between organisations, cultures, systems, geographical areas and resources can be considerable and therefore a barrier to collaboration. It can be difficult to convene groups of professionals owing to the demands of respective services. Indeed it can be very expensive for multidisciplinary groups to meet at the same time. It is not unusual for there to be low levels of *Interdisciplinary working* because no one agency will take a lead responsibility.

Provided that there are clear reasons, educationalists are well positioned to coordinate interdisciplinary working. The disadvantage of this can be the attendant work in organisation, such as providing minutes and chasing up agreements. The way in which joint working is organised and agreed can impose various constraints depending on the specific arrangements put into place.

Where interdisciplinary meetings (Figure 1) are needed, the following pointers are worth considering:

- Be clear about the purposes and benefits for the child and for all services with all participants.

- Liaise with parents to explore if any duplicate meetings can be avoided. Could an existing meeting be transformed into a multidisciplinary meeting?
- Develop an understanding of 'better times' for key colleagues to meet.
- Be flexible about where to meet.
- Be absolutely clear of the intentions of the meeting; express the common vision – set these out in the agenda showing where the advice and input from other professionals is necessary.
- Do not ask people to meetings with a specific focus if it does not require their input. Accurate minutes will keep other team members up to date.
- Create a folder such as a ring file in which parents can keep their copies of plans and minutes. Provide a multidisciplinary 'diary' such as a ring file for visiting professionals. (See Figure 2.)
- Document outcomes, setting out expectations explicitly for others, and set timelines for work.
- It may be possible for agencies to take turns to coordinate, organise and host meetings.
- Structures and hierarchies differ; decisions from some colleagues might have to be agreed through line management and/or committees – where this is the case, plan ahead to avoid putting people under pressure.
- It is a good idea to combine an Annual Review of a Statement or an internal school review with an interdisciplinary meeting.

Working together in combinations that are required to support a child in school can take

The next meeting of the multidisciplinary team will take place at <Time> < Venue>

INFORMATION ABOUT THE CHILD

Name	
DOB	
Address	
Special Educational Needs	
School	
Health Centre	

PARENTS' or CARER'S INFORMATION

Names	
Address	
Telephone	
Access Information	

DETAILS of FAMILY

Figure 1a Samples of interdisciplinary meeting papers: Information Sheet for Multidisciplinary Meeting

MULTI-AGENCY TEAM CONTACT INFORMATION

The child's needs determine the different professionals required to constitute an effective team. Preferred contact arrangements will need to be mutually agreed.

Contributor	Name	Contact address	Telephone	E-mail
Team Coordinator				
Parent/s Carers				
Class Teacher				
LSA				
Physiotherapist				
Occupational Therapist				
Speech and Language Therapist				
School Medical Officer				
School Nurse				
Social Worker				
Specialist or Family Health Visitor				
Specialist Teacher				
Educational Psychologist				
General Practitioner				
Consultant(s)				
Key-worker				

Figure 1b Samples of interdisciplinary meeting papers: Multi-Agency Team Contact

WHAT	WHO	WHEN

Figure 1c Sample of interdisciplinary meeting papers: Action Plan

ACTION TAKEN SINCE LAST MEETING BY VISITING PROFESSIONALS

WHO	WHEN	WHAT

Figure 2 Sample of transdisciplinary diary

careful planning. Those working in schools should consider the following:

- Where the school is the focus of the interdisciplinary working, ensure that time for release to do the work is built into the timetable of the teacher, the SENCO or Learning Support Assistant. Time to collaborate and to talk is time well spent as it is not easy to establish clarification or discuss important matters while in class.
- Be sensitive to the constraints on other professionals by their service. Effective use of time means people will try to cluster or group their work in geographical areas as they might have more than one child to see in a school or within a locality of schools.
- Help and encourage colleagues to see the child at the same time if that is beneficial. For example where physical positioning and a particular piece of equipment are being changed and reviewed, it is good for the physiotherapist, occupational therapist and equipment provider to be with the child at the same time. Similarly, where a child is using a speech output device, the Speech and Language Therapist, Assisted Communication Teacher and Hearing Impaired Teacher could usefully collaborate with child and parents in determining the next steps in a communication programme.
- Where collaborative working becomes difficult, make arrangements for necessary communications to be the responsibility of each professional. Avoid becoming the 'messenger' for others as details of an unfamiliar area of work can easily be misunderstood or distorted. The best arrangement is to have a transdisciplinary diary – a loose-leaf format is sensible where each professional can leave their written advice or questions for other members of the team.
- Provide all members of the team with a contact sheet giving the information needed in order to make contacts together with an up-to-date plan. Sometimes it is worth knowing the timetables of peripatetic teaching staff, as in this way contact could be made at other schools.

Key publications information

Worthington, A. (ed.). *The Fulton Special Education Digest*. London: David Fulton, 1999, Section 2, pp. 21–34.

Key contact information

National Association of Special Educational Needs (NASEN)
NASEN House
4/5 Amber Business Village
Amber Close
Amington
Tamworth B77 4RP
Tel: 01827 311500
E-mail: welcome@nasen.org.uk
www.nasen.org.uk

The SENCO Electronic Communication Project
www.becta.org.uk/inclusion/senco/
Senco-forum Mailing List Archive
http://forum.ngfl.gov.uk/senco-forum/

4 A–Z entries

Throughout this section, cross-references to other conditions are given in italics. References to *Interdisciplinary working* refer to the last section in the previous chapter.

A

Abdominal migraine

Abdominal migraine consists of recurrent episodes of abdominal pain, nausea, occasional vomiting and visual disturbance. Episodes are usually terminated when the child falls asleep and awakes without symptoms. There is often a family history of migraine. Treatments include pain relief and medication to try and prevent attacks.

Children with abdominal migraine can have their educational needs met in mainstream and special schools. School-based *Interdisciplinary working* might be necessary for some children, while community medical services will manage others. Effective links with parents and good pastoral arrangements will provide support for these children.

Possible causes of abdominal migraine including stress, fatigue and exertion should be considered and where possible be avoided. At times some children may find temporary access to a quiet room helpful. Although the school day might at times be disrupted, it is unlikely that the curriculum should be modified for children because they have abdominal migraine.

Useful links
The Migraine Trust
45 Great Ormond Street
London WC1N 3HZ
Tel: 020 7831 4818
www.migrainetrust.org

Abdominal pain

Abdominal pain can be caused by most of the conditions that affect the gut, including inflammation and infection of any of its contents. Pains indicative of particular illnesses or conditions tend to have specific patterns and sites in the abdomen. For example, children with oesophagitis (inflamed gullet) can have heartburn or chest pain.

In functional abdominal pain, children

have recurring painful episodes for which no underlying condition or diagnosis can be found, despite (in some cases) extensive tests. Reasons may therefore be psychosocial. The pains are typically centred around the umbilicus (tummy button), and rarely cause diarrhoea or vomiting. In some children, recurrent abdominal pains may be a form of migraine (*Abdominal migraine*). In others, pain in the tummy may be a reaction to stress or anxiety. Treatment is symptomatic, following reassurance that the pains do not represent any serious problem with the bowel or other abdominal contents. Addressing the ongoing causes of stress in such children is usually the most rewarding line of management.

Most schools have children who at some time will have abdominal pain. Effective links with parents and good pastoral arrangements will provide support for these children. The school cannot ignore the child in distress and arrangements to return home might need to be made. Absence may need careful monitoring.

Achondroplasia

Achondroplasia is an inherited condition (although many children have no family history of achondroplasia), whereby the bones stop growing early on in life, severely limiting the height of the affected child. It can also lead to bony abnormalities of the skull and spine. Some children might have their condition complicated by *Hydrocephalus*. The early motor milestones of sitting up, crawling and walking could be delayed. For the affected child, short stature brings social and emotional problems.

Children with achondroplasia can be educated in mainstream and special schools. The extent to which this condition affects schooling depends on the child's size and whether medical interventions are required. School-based *Interdisciplinary working* involving a physiotherapist and an occupational therapist might be necessary for some children; community medical services will manage others. Effective links with parents and good pastoral arrangements will provide support for children.

Children with achondroplasia need access to the same curriculum as their peers. Special attention might be needed to gross and fine motor development and speech and language development. It will be important to give careful consideration to all aspects of being physically smaller than everyone else in a school (see *Physical disability* and *Disfigurement and difference*). If a child moves school, it is important to audit and take action in sufficient time for changes and planning to be in place. Can external and internal doors be easily opened? Are coat hooks, toilets, sinks, soap dispensers, towels accessible? Are corridors and stairs safe? Pay attention to lunchtime arrangements and playtimes. A good way of carrying out this work is to ask parents and the occupational therapist who knows the child to walk through the school. In the classroom, adapted furniture may be needed to provide correct posture, comfort and curricular access. Scissors, pencils and pens and other standard learning implements may need adapting. Ensure that the smaller child has the same access to PE and physical activities as their peers. When school and residential trips are organised, plan well ahead and, if you are travelling by road, check seat belts or safety restraints.

Useful links
Restricted Growth Association
PO Box 4744
Dorchester DT2 9FA
Tel: 01308 898445
E-mail: rga1@talk21.com
www.rgaonline.org.uk

Achromatopsia

Achromatopsia is a condition affecting the centre of the retina causing either total or almost total colour blindness, and poor visual acuity.

Children with achromatopsia can be educated in mainstream and special schools. The extent to which this condition affects schooling will depend on the severity of colour blindness and visual acuity. School-based *Interdisciplinary working* involving a specialist teacher for visual impairment might be necessary for some children; community medical services will manage others. Effective links with parents and good pastoral arrangements will provide support for these children.

Problems with vision may affect development of movement, coordination and speech. For further information see *Visual impairment*.

Useful links
NOAH (The National Organization for Albinism and Hypopigmentation)
PO Box 959
East Hampstead
NH 03826-0959

USA
Tel: 001 800 473 2310
Tel/Fax: 001 603 887 2310
E-mail: webmaster@albinism.org
www.albinism.org

RNIB Education Information Services
224 Great Portland Street
London W1N 6AA
Tel: 020 7388 1266
www.rnib.org.uk

Acne

Acne occurs in many youngsters as they go through puberty. The hormonal changes cause glands in the skin to secrete a fatty substance called sebum. This blocks the gland and inflammation and infection follows. Most cases are mild. Some children are more severely affected and might require medication either directly on the skin or occasionally by mouth. Good information from the school nurse and an effective pastoral system will usually provide the support needed. The curriculum will not need to be modified for children because they have acne.

For some children even mild acne can have social and psychological effects. Staff in school can do a number of things to help, including watching for cruel taunts, embarrassment and lack of eye contact, growing hair long to cover the face, and looking for those pupils who avoid socialising and become withdrawn. Careful sympathetic support will go a long way with some pupils. Treat pupils who taunt and bully according to school policy. Some youngsters will avoid doing sport because of the need to remove clothes in changing rooms. In extreme circumstances pupils can become significantly depressed and experience loss of appetite, lethargy, mood changes, wakefulness and feelings of unworthiness; this, in turn, can affect school performance. In these cases, it is most important to work closely with home and possibly seek expert counselling.

Useful links
The Acne Support Group
PO Box 230
Hayes B4 0UT
Tel: 020 8561 6868
www.m2w3.com/acne/

Acne Support Group
Howard House
The Runway
South Ruislip A4 6SE
Tel: 020 8841 4747
www.stopspots.org/

British Association of Dermatologists
19 Fitzroy Square
London W1T 6EH
Tel: 020 7383 0266
Fax: 020 7388 5263
E-mail: admin@bad.org.uk
www.skinhealth.co.uk/contact/index.htm

Adjustment disorder

Children with adjustment disorder develop temporary affective (emotional) or behavioural symptoms in response to a known source. Sources can include natural disasters, events or crises such as car accidents or sudden severe illness, or interpersonal problems such as family breakdown or abuse. Children display distress and are unable to work or study. Adjustment disorders, by definition, last less than six months after the original cause or its consequences end. If the symptoms last for more than six months, the child might have another disorder, such as an anxiety or mood disorder.

The temporary nature of this condition will mean that staff in school should be aware of the children's particular anxiety, distress or vulnerability. A whole-school approach, with pastoral support and attention to the demands of the curriculum, will help support these children. Good parental liaison is essential especially in cases where physical violence has been experienced. The support of external specialists may be helpful (see *Interdisciplinary working*).

Adrenoleukodystrophies *see* Leukodystrophies

Agenesis of the corpus callosum

Agenesis of the corpus callosum is a congenital condition whereby the middle part of the brain that connects the two hemispheres has not formed completely. This can result in a range of problems. In some children it causes no difficulties at all, but in others it can cause epilepsy, learning difficulties, visiospatial difficulties, and other problems with the formation of centrally placed organs such as the heart, main arteries, genitals and some hormone-producing glands.

School-based *Interdisciplinary working* involving a physiotherapist, an occupational therapist and a speech and language therapist might be necessary for some children, while community medical services will manage others. Effective links with parents and good pastoral arrangements will provide support for these children.

Children with agenesis of the corpus callosum will generally experience severe and complex learning disability requiring a highly differentiated curriculum (see *Physical disability*, *Epilepsy* and *Visual impairment*). Children with agenesis of the corpus callosum will need access to the same curriculum as their peers.

Useful links
CORPAL
240 Malden Way
New Malden KT3 5QU
Tel: 020 8404 6620
E-mail: corpal@blueyonder.co.uk
www.corpal.org.uk

AIDS *see* Human immunodeficiency virus

Albinism

Albinism causes a deficiency of the pigment known as melanin (present in the skin and eyes). When the eyes are affected, the condition is known as ocular albinism. Here there is a lack of melanin pigment at the back of the eye and in the iris. This can lead to poor vision, a dislike of bright light and difficulties with eye movement (see *Nystagmus*). Treatment consists of correcting any long- or short-sightedness and providing tinted glasses to reduce the amount of light entering the eye.

Albinism can result in the child being partially sighted. For further advice see *Visual impairment*. Children with albinism can be educated in mainstream and special schools. School-based *Interdisciplinary working* will be necessary, including the advice of a specialist teacher for visual impairment in the planning of an effective educational programme. Teachers will need to consider where the child will sit in the classroom, and use of large print, optical aids and non-optical aids. Access to the curriculum should be modified for children because they have albinism.

Useful links
NOAH
The National Organization for Albinism and Hypopigmentation
PO Box 959
East Hampstead
NH 03826-0959
USA
Tel: 001 800 473 2310
Tel/Fax: 001 603 887 2310
E-mail: webmaster@albinism.org
www.albinism.org
NOAH is a volunteer organisation for persons and families involved with the condition of albinism. It does not diagnose or treat, or provide genetic counselling. It is involved in self-help, while trying to promote research and education.

Hands and Eyes
A USA specialist teacher maintains this useful online newsletter for teachers and caregivers of visually impaired students and their friends. It includes art, cooking and manipulative activities that visually impaired students can do individually or in small groups. It is for teachers and support staff in need of ideas for classroom activities and is particularly useful for pupils with multiple impairments such as developmental disability and motor impairment.
www.home.earthlink.net/~vharris/

RNIB Education Information Services
224 Great Portland Street
London W1N 6AA
Tel: 020 7388 1266
E-mail: webmaster@rnib.org.uk
www.rnib.org.uk
RNIB's curriculum information service offers information and advice to all professionals supporting a visually impaired child in mainstream or special schools.
www.rnib.org.uk/curriculum/
RNIB's accessing technology pages provide information about applications of technology in employment, at study and in leisure.
www.rnib.org.uk/technology/

V.I. Guide
This site contains information on many topics relating to parenting and teaching a child with visual impairments.
www.viguide.com/

Albright's hereditary osteodystrophy

Albright's hereditary osteodystrophy is a rare condition. Affected children have obesity, bony lumps under the skin and sometimes learning difficulties. It is in part due to difficulties in maintaining the correct level of calcium in the child.

Children with Albright's hereditary osteodystrophy can be educated in mainstream and special schools. The extent to which this condition affects schooling depends on the medical interventions required. Most children will have their condition managed by community medical services. Effective links with parents and good pastoral arrangements will provide support for these children. It is unlikely that the curriculum should be modified for children because they have Albright's hereditary osteodystrophy.

Useful links
Climb
The Quadrangle
Crewe Hall, Weston Road
Crewe CW2 6UR
Tel: 0870 770 0326
E-mail: info@climb.org.uk
www.climb.org.uk

Alexia

Alexia is the loss of a previously acquired ability to read owing to disease or injury to the brain, and it is distinct from *Dyslexia* (see also *Speech disorder*).

Alternative and augmentative communication (AAC)

AAC is the collective term used to refer to techniques or aids that add meaning to, or are used instead of, speech. AAC is an area of multidisciplinary practice working to make temporary or permanent arrangements for those impairments and disabilities in individuals who have severe expressive communication disorders. Arrangements can range from simple non-technological aids through to the most sophisticated equipment and arrangements that technology can provide.

Children who are not communicating for

any reason will be subject to review by professionals inside and outside school. A proposal for a communication assessment should be made carefully with parents through well-informed *Interdisciplinary working*. The key professionals should include a speech and language therapist specialising in AAC, a specialist teacher for communication, and an educational psychologist. Where children have physical difficulties, then a physiotherapist and an occupational therapist should be involved. Different arrangements for assessment will exist in different localities. If the education department does not have an agreed route for referral, then a multidisciplinary assessment should be requested from elsewhere; for example at one of the ACE Centres and more recently through the CAP Project (Communications Aids Project) managed by Becta.

Before assessments take place, the team generally require detailed reports and a video of the child in his or her own setting. At the assessment, it is best practice to arrange for parents and all those professionally involved to attend along with the child. In this way the assessing team are most likely to elicit the information that they need to make well-informed judgements. In some circumstances the assessing team will do the assessment in the child's school or home. Following the assessment, a detailed report together with recommendations is sent to the referring agency. Where the school or education department has made the referral, then the recommendations should be implemented within the approved procedures. Some equipment can be very expensive and its purchase can be subject to long bureau-

cratic procedure. It is important that children do not wait for months for the means to communicate and to participate.

There are generally three broad types of alternative and augmentative communication:

No tech

The range of 'no tech' communication can only be limited by the imagination of those concerned. At a very simple level there is the ability to express likes or dislikes by pointing in some way to something that indicates either YES or NO. Pointing can be done with eyes, limbs or a device held or attached to a part of the body over which the child has consistent voluntary control. In this way children can make choices and begin to have a degree of control over their environment.

Manual signing systems such as British Sign Language (BSL) and MAKATON are used extensively with children who need a means of expression. MAKATON is a vocabulary derived from the BSL and uses signs that are symbolic and not necessarily dependant on spelling or syntax. Users of BSL will sign with much greater specificity, using finger spelling to make the words they need. Signing must always be accompanied by speech. Where signing is the prime means of communication, it is likely that children are going to be educated in specialist settings where there will be a signing environment, possibly in the context of a total communication policy. Greater inclusion will mean that all schools will have an increasing experience of children who are using signing to support their communication.

Low tech

There are a variety of simple devices available to store speech or simple messages. These can then be used to give children the message or words that they need in certain settings. Usually these can be switch-operated provided that the child has some voluntary muscular control. Children will start using switches to activate devices that store speech. A 'BIGMACK' is a large easily used cylindrical device that can store a single word or a short phrase and is triggered by the integral switch or through an externally connected switch. These simple devices can be used for special activities such as answering the register, participating in stories or taking messages to other teachers.

There are other simple devices that will store two, four or eight messages – these can be used with multiple switches giving the child an increased vocabulary. Most schools will be able to access advice on the use of these through their speech and language therapist or their local special school. The use and positioning of switches is likely to involve the physiotherapist and occupational therapist.

High tech

These more complex devices will generally be available following a multidisciplinary assessment in which case arrangements for the training of staff concerned and the longer term maintenance and eventual upgrade of the equipment should be planned. Sophisticated speech output devices are usually specially adapted portable computers that can store vast vocabularies, different voices, and can be worked through a touch-screen or a range of external peripherals. Most devices can be set up for scanning, where a single switch is used, and pictures are highlighted in sequence either visually or using sound. When the desired picture is highlighted, the user activates it by pressing or releasing the switch.

Alternative and augmentative communication is a rapidly growing aspect of special education, attracting increasing attention from central government and local education authorities.

Useful links
ACE Centre – North
1 Broadbent Road
Watersheddings
Oldham
Greater Manchester OL1 4HU
Tel: 0161 627 1358
E-mail: acenorth@ace-north.org.uk
www.ace-north.org.uk
The ACE Centre – North offers independent interdisciplinary services to enable the effective use of assistive technology for individuals with physical and communications impairments. Services include assessments, training advice, professional development, information and consultancy, and help for parents. The centre is funded by Oldham MBC, Becta and generated income. The assessment team consists of teachers, speech and language therapists and occupational therapists.

ACE Centre Advisory Trust
92 Windmill Road
Headington
Oxford OX3 7DR
Tel: 01865 759800
E-mail: info@ace-centre.org.uk
www.ace-centre.org.uk

The ACE (Aids to Communication in Education) Centre in Oxford provides a focus of information and experience in relation to the use of microelectronics as an aid to communication. Its services and facilities include detailed assessments of individuals, and software development and multidisciplinary training. The ACE Centre produces a series of guides to software, switches and equipment to support those with communication difficulties, and is actively involved in training and research. Their staff provide advice and there is a telephone helpline.

Becta
Tel: 024 7684 7113
www.becta.org.uk/news/index.htm
Becta is the Government's lead agency for ICT in education. Becta supports the UK Government and national organisations in the use and development of ICT in education to raise standards, widen access, improve skills and encourage effective management.

Centre for Micro-Assisted Communication (CENMAC)
Charlton Park School
Charlton Park Road
London SE7 8JB
Tel: 020 8854 1019
E-mail: cenmac@cenmac.greenwich.gov.uk
www.cenmac.demon.co.uk
The Centre for Micro-Assisted Communication provides assessment and support for children with communication difficulties caused by physical difficulties. It covers the Inner London area and collaborates with SENJIT to provide training opportunities for the South East England region. It also offers training and information and undertakes private assessments and consultancy to schools and colleges.

The Communication Aids for Language and Learning (CALL) Centre
University of Edinburgh
Patersons Lane
Holyrood Road
Edinburgh EH8 8AQ
Tel: 0131 651 6235
E-mail: call-centre@ed.ac.uk
http://callcentre.education.ed.ac.uk
The CALL centre provides services and carries out research and development projects, working with all those involved in meeting the special needs of people who require augmentative communication and/or specialised technology use, particularly in education. Primarily, the Scottish Office Education and Industry Department and social work service group funds CALL.

Communication Matters
c/o ACE Centre
93 Windmill Road
Headington
Oxford OX3 7DR
Tel: 0870 606 5463
E-mail: admin@communicationmatters.org.uk
www.communicationmatters.org.uk
Communication Matters is a UK voluntary organisation focusing on the needs of people with severe communication difficulties who might benefit from AAC systems to maximise their opportunities and enhance their life.

Providers of AAC equipment:
Assistive Technology:
www.assistivetech.com/
Communication Devices, Inc:
www.comdevices.com
Dyna Vox Systems Inc:
www.dynavoxsys.com

Gus Communications, Inc:
www.gusinc.com
Toby Churchill, Ltd:
www.toby-churchill.demon.co.uk

Ambiguous genitalia

Ambiguous genitalia is the term for genitals that are not obviously male or female. It is caused by enzyme deficiencies or other genetic or chemical problems, which result in abnormal formation of the genital tissue. It can also be associated with abnormalities of the urinary system (see *Hypospadias*). Some children can have other problems associated with the condition, for example salt imbalance, requiring medication. Children with female chromosomes might have male type genitalia and vice versa. Treatment can be with medications and/or surgery; psychological support will be required as these children can have great difficulties with their sexual identity as they grow up.

Children with ambiguous genitalia can be educated in mainstream and special schools. Generally children will have their condition attended to by community medical services. Children and young people may need counselling relating to the development of gender identity; this work is usually carried out by skilled teams and, on rare occasions, might involve staff in school. Effective links with parents and good pastoral arrangements will provide support for these children.

Where staff are aware that children have been or are undergoing treatment for ambiguous genitalia, then situations where their differences may become evident, such as changing rooms and shared accommodation on school trips and residentials, must be considered carefully. As this may be a matter of confidentiality, key staff will need to develop ways of monitoring children to prevent inappropriate comments and/or bullying. It is unlikely that the curriculum should be significantly modified for these children.

Useful links
The United Kingdom Intersex Association (UKIA)
E-mail: jhl@ukia.co.uk
www.ukia.co.uk

Anaemia

Anaemia occurs when the amount of haemoglobin in the blood is reduced. Haemoglobin is the molecule responsible for the red colour of blood and transports oxygen from the lungs around the body. Most anaemia is dietary in origin and caused by lack of iron. Supplements can be given or an iron-rich diet might be recommended. Other sorts of anaemia might be due to other long-term illnesses requiring their own specific treatments. It is thought by many doctors that very young anaemic children do not learn as well as children without anaemia because iron is needed for brain development.

Children with anaemia can be educated in mainstream and special schools. School-based *Interdisciplinary working* might be necessary for some children, while community medical services will manage others. Some children may need to take medication during the school day. Others might need food intake to be monitored because of special dietary requirements. Some children can experience fatigue and have limited stamina; otherwise it is unlikely that any curriculum adaptations are needed. Good pastoral systems are useful to provide support and in some cases counselling.

Anaphylaxis

Anaphylaxis is a violent and severe allergic reaction to a commonplace substance or food – for instance, peanuts. The child's immune system recognises the substance and reacts by releasing a chemical called histamine. This can cause the child's airway tissues to swell, wheezing, a fast heart rate, sweating, low blood pressure and unconsciousness. Children will have had a past episode of a severe reaction, usually to an identified substance or food. Treatment is avoidance of the trigger substance, and severely affected children might be issued with an automatic adrenaline injector, for example an Epi-pen, to be used in the event of an attack.

Children with anaphylaxis can be educated in mainstream and special schools. The extent to which anaphylaxis affects schooling depends on the allergies affecting the children. This condition is usually simply managed by community medical services. *Interdisciplinary working* is useful for determining a protocol or agreement and any training needs concerning the use of an Epi-pen. Effective links with parents and good pastoral arrangements might be needed.

Children with anaphylaxis should not need different curriculum arrangements. All staff will need to know what needs to be done in the event of a situation requiring the use of an Epi-pen and the possibility of a hospital visit. Affected children should be encouraged to have a 'crisis plan' that is made known to their friends and to staff in school. School trips/visits and residential outings will need careful planning.

Affected children will know what to avoid and will usually be good at avoiding the substance or food that causes the allergic reaction. Whatever measures a school takes to protect affected children, staff and parents will need to maintain continuous vigilance. The best plans can simply be undone through ignorance or lack of communication. There are many things a school can consider, including being a nut-free zone, not passing round sweets on birthdays, systems for vetting all foodstuffs/substances that enter the school, encouraging children to read food labels and the labels of other products, making sure that all staff know what to do and that new staff are informed.

Useful links
Action against Allergy
PO Box 278
Twickenham TW1 4QQ
Tel: 020 8892 2711
E-mail:
AAA@actionagainstallergy.freeserve.co.uk
www.actionagainstallergy.co.uk

The Anaphylaxis Campaign
PO Box 275

Farnborough GU14 7SX

Tel: 01252 542029

E-mail: anaphylaxis.campaign@virgin.net

www.anaphylaxis.org.uk.

Breathe Easy

British Lung Foundation

78 Hatton Garden

London EC1N 8LD

Tel: 020 7831 5831

E-mail: blf@britishlungfoundation.com

www.lunguk.org

British Allergy Foundation

Deepdene House

30 Bellegrove Road

Welling DA16 3PY

Tel: 020 8303 8583

E-mail: info@allergyfoundation.com

www.allergyfoundation.com

DfES Publications Centre

PO Box 5050

Sudbury CO10 6ZQ

Tel: 0845 602 2260

www.dfes.gov.uk/medical/

Supporting Pupils With Medical Needs – A Good Practice Guide. *This is a document to help schools draw up policies on managing medication in schools, and to put in place effective management systems to support individual pupils with medical needs. It can be downloaded from the DfES website.*

National Society for Research into Allergies and Environmental Diseases

PO Box 45

Hinckley LE10 1JY

Tel/Fax: 01455 250715

E-mail: nsra.allergy@virgin.net

Angelman syndrome

Angelman syndrome is a rare condition that causes a child to have severe learning difficulties, epilepsy, speech problems, unsteady walking and other movement problems. It is caused when the child inherits faulty copies of part of chromosome 15 with loss of genetic material. Children with Angelman syndrome have delayed walking, and when this is finally achieved, it is often unsteady. They are also emotionally labile and can seem inappropriately happy or sad.

Children with Angelman syndrome have severe or profound learning difficulties and will need a highly differentiated curriculum. School-based *Interdisciplinary working* is essential and should include therapists, specialist teachers and educational psychologists in order to design the most appropriate educational programme.

Some children will have a range of physical difficulties (see *Physical disability*). *Verbal dyspraxia* and *Dyspraxia* is common together with overactivity. Significant attention should be given to communication, as many children will have little or no spoken language. A communication programme should be devised together with a speech and language therapist. This might include the use of gestures, signing, symbols and picture systems. Some children will benefit from *Alternative and augmentative communication* devices.

As a feature of Angelman syndrome is emotional lability, some children can display quite challenging behaviours that can disrupt a class. Some children can be very excitable and benefit from low arousal techniques based on careful observation and a good knowledge of what might trigger or stimulate the child. As many have short concentration spans, it is a good idea to have a number of different relevant activities ready within each session to hold the child's attention.

Useful links
Angelman Syndrome Support Group
15 Place Crescent
Waterlooville
Portsmouth PO7 5UR
Tel: 023 9226 4224

ASSERT
PO Box 505
Sittingbourne ME10 1NE
Tel: 01980 652617
E-mail: assert@dial.pipex.com
www.assert.dial.pipex.com

Anophthalmia

Anophthalmia means the absence of the eye. It usually occurs as a congenital defect, which means that the baby is born with the condition. The other eye might be affected, either partially or fully. Other defects of the face or central nervous system can also occur, meaning that these children have other difficulties in addition to the obvious visual problems.

Children with anophthalmia can be educated in mainstream and special schools. Some children may have prosthetic eyes fitted and this can lead to medical management issues. School-based *Interdisciplinary working* might be necessary for some children, while community medical services will manage others. For further advice see *Visual impairment* and *Blindness*. If the child's

appearance is adversely affected, see *Disfigurement and difference*. Generally, children with anophthalmia need a highly specialised curriculum.

Useful links
The Micro & Anophthalmic Childrens Society
1 Skyrmans
Frinton on Sea CO13 0RN
Tel/Fax: 01255 677511
E-mail: macs.uk@btinternet.com
www.macs.org.uk

RNIB Education Information Services
224 Great Portland Street
London W1N 6AA
Tel: 020 7388 1266
E-mail: webmaster@rnib.org.uk
www.rnib.org.uk
RNIB's curriculum information service offers information and advice to all professionals supporting a visually impaired child in mainstream or special schools.
www.rnib.org.uk/curriculum/
RNIB's accessing technology pages provide information about applications of technology in employment, at study and in leisure.
www.rnib.org.uk/technology/

Hands and Eyes
A USA specialist teacher maintains this useful online newsletter for teachers and caregivers of visually impaired students and their friends. It includes art, cooking and manipulative activities that visually impaired students can do individually or in small groups. It is for teachers and support staff in need of ideas for classroom activities and is particularly useful for pupils with multiple impairments such as developmental disability and motor impairment.
www.home.earthlink.net/~vharris/

V.I. Guide

This site contains information on many topics relating to parenting and teaching a child with visual impairments.

www.viguide.com/

Anorexia nervosa

Anorexia nervosa is an illness that usually occurs in teenage girls, but it can also occur in boys. Children and young people with anorexia are obsessed with being thin. They lose a lot of weight and are terrified of becoming overweight. They develop a distorted body image and believe they are fat even though they are very thin. It is thought that children with anorexia attempt to use food and weight to deal with emotional and psychological problems.

Where children have eating disorders, it is necessary to work closely with the family and the wider multidisciplinary team (see *Interdisciplinary working*). The school's pastoral systems will be needed to support the child to help manage their condition. It is important to make sure that support mechanisms extend beyond the classroom.

Useful links
ABC
PO Box 30
Ormskirk L39 5JR
Tel: 01695 422479
E-mail:
doreen@AnorexiaBulimiaCare.co.uk
www.anorexiabulimiacare.co.uk

Eating Disorders Association
103 Prince of Wales Road

Norwich NR1 1DW
Tel: 01603 621414
E-mail: info@edauk.com
www.edauk.com/

Anotia

Anotia is the absence of the pinna, the external ear. It is usually congenital and the child is born with the problem. It might also be associated with absence or abnormal development of the middle or inner ear and, in some cases, can be bilateral. It is a rare condition, often associated with other abnormalities of the face or skull. Where the outside of the ear is abnormally small, which is often due to similar congenital problems, the child is said to have microtia. Treatment varies. If the remaining ear has good hearing, then the condition poses cosmetic difficulties whereas, when both ears are affected, specialised hearing aids (such as bone-anchored devices) might be required.

For the child with these conditions, hearing, communication and cosmetic difficulties predominate. This physical omission will mean the children's educational provision will be interrupted while restorative surgery takes place. Advances in tissue 'engineering' might mean children spending considerable periods of time under close medical supervision. Some children might have a *Cochlear implant* and need the additional specialised support to learn how to use the aid. Medical interventions may be at an advanced stage by the time the chid is in preschool provision or attending their first primary school.

Children with anotia can be educated in mainstream and special schools. School-based *Interdisciplinary working* involving specialist teachers, audiologists and audio technicians might be necessary for some children, while others will have their condition managed by hospital or community medical services. Effective links with parents and good pastoral arrangements will provide support for these children. For further information see *Hearing impairment*. Children needing frequent absence from school and time-consuming treatments can lead staff to have low expectations and disrupt school friendships. It is important to explore all possible ways of supporting children who are absent for long periods and to provide a range of ways to help them catch up with work; this becomes very important where children are mid-syllabus for externally accredited examinations. Children might need medication during the school day in which case school policy and procedures on the administration of medication should be followed.

Apert's syndrome

Apert's syndrome affects the development of the head, face and hands. The skull bones can fuse early on during development causing an abnormal head shape, while the eye sockets are often shallow making the eyes protuberant. The fingers of the hand might be fused together and the thumbs might be abnormal. Some children might have associated developmental and learning difficulties (which can be severe), while others are not affected. Children may have undergone surgery to the face, head and hands already or surgery might be planned during the child's time in education. The affected child might have to cope with reactions from others to such facial problems and possibly to difficulties with manipulation, as well as any learning difficulty.

Children with Apert's syndrome can be educated in mainstream schools and special schools. The extent to which Apert's syndrome affects schooling depends on the ways in which the symptoms present themselves and the consequent medical interventions required. School-based *Interdisciplinary working* including the advice of specialist teachers, therapists and possibly educational psychologist might be necessary for some children, while community medical services will manage others. Effective links with parents and good pastoral arrangements will provide support for these children. When surgery is needed children can be educated by the hospital school or service; it is very important to have good effective channels of communication between the child's local school and hospital school in order to provide continuity of curriculum.

For some children their differences have social and psychological effects. Staff in school can do a number of things to help, including watching for cruel taunts, playground unpleasantness, social avoidance and withdrawal (see *Disfigurement and difference*). Children with Apert's syndrome will need access to the same curriculum as their peers; however, some modification might be needed because of impaired vision and hearing. Some children's fine motor skills can be affected and special assistance may be needed particularly with holding pencils, pens, scissors and other instruments.

Useful links
Changing Faces
1 & 2 Junction Mews

London W2 1PN
Tel: 020 7706 4232
E-mail: info@changingfaces.co.uk
www.cfaces.demon.co.uk

The Disfigurement Guidance Centre
PO Box 7
Cupar
Fife KY15 4PF
www.dgc.org.uk

Aphasia

Aphasia is a speech disorder originating in the central nervous system after language acquisition is complete; this can be caused by brain disease or physical damage to the brain, damage from strokes, trauma, epilepsy or sometimes infectious disease (see *Speech disorder*).

Aplasia cutis

Aplasia cutis appears in newborns as areas of skin that have failed to develop. These areas are usually small and occur in the middle of the scalp, although they can occur elsewhere. Treatment can include surgery.

Children with aplasia cutis can be educated in mainstream and special schools. The extent to which aplasia cutis affects schooling depends on the medical interventions required. School-based *Interdisciplinary working* might be necessary for some children, while community medical services will manage others. The curriculum will not need to be modified because children have aplasia cutis.

Useful links
British Association of Dermatologists

19 Fitzroy Square
London W1T 6EH
Tel: 020 7383 0266
Fax: 020 7388 5263
E-mail: admin@bad.org.uk
www.skinhealth.co.uk/contact/index.htm

Appendicitis

Some children can develop characteristic abdominal pains, fever and other symptoms that suggest the appendix is inflamed. The appendix is a small redundant piece of bowel that becomes inflamed in some children for obscure reasons. Treatment is by surgical removal. Other children might also have episodes of fever and abdominal pain owing to the inflammation of lymph glands in the abdomen. It may accompany sore throats or ear infections. These symptoms can closely mimic those of appendicitis. Treatment is for the pain and fever.

Children who have appendicitis will at some point need surgery. Some children can be educated temporarily through the hospital education service or school; others will quickly return to school.

Arteritis

Arteritis is the term given to inflamed blood vessels. It occurs in conditions such as *Henoch–Schönlein purpura*, *Dermatomyositis*, *Juvenile arthritis* and *Systemic lupus erythamatosus* (see individual entries for details).

Children with arteritis can be educated in mainstream and special schools. The extent to which arteritis affects schooling depends on the medical interventions required. School-based *Interdisciplinary working* might be necessary for some children, while community medical services will manage others. Effective links with parents and good pastoral arrangements will provide the child with physical and emotional support.

Children with arteritis will need access to the same curriculum as their peers. Special arrangements will probably be needed to provide access to physically demanding sporting activities including a place to rest when or if tired. The safety measures for all pupils are generally sufficient. Overall children with arteritis have a condition that from time to time can interfere with their education.

Arthritis

Arthritis is damage to, or, disease of a joint or joints. The child can experience pain, swelling and loss of joint function. This in turn can affect mobility, manipulation and self-care. Treatment is to try and reduce pain and swelling. There are a number of different forms of arthritis affecting children.

Children with arthritis can be educated in mainstream and special schools. The extent to which this condition affects schooling depends on severity of the condition and the medical interventions required. For some children pain management is important; others might experience long periods of restricted mobility and will need exercises designed by a physiotherapist. School-based *Interdisciplinary working* involving a physiotherapist and an occupational therapist might be necessary for some children, while others will have their condition managed by community

medical services. Effective links with parents and good pastoral arrangements will provide support for these children.

Children with arthritis will need access to the same curriculum as their peers. Children in the primary phase may need special attention – they might not tell staff when they are in discomfort or have a problem, because they are engrossed in a particular activity or because they might prefer to avoid treatment. Some children will need wheelchairs – therefore access to classrooms and the building needs to be good (see *Physical disability*). Advice from medical professionals might be needed to ensure that exercises, activities and games in PE are appropriate. Overall children with arthritis have a condition that can sometimes interfere with their education.

Useful links
Arthritis Care Youth Service
The Source
18 Stephenson Way
London NW1 2HD
Tel: 0808 808 2000
E-mail: thesource@arthritiscare.org.uk
www.arthritiscare.org.uk

Children's Chronic Arthritis Association
Ground Floor Office, Amber Gate
City Walls Road
Worcester WR1 2AH
Tel: 01905 745595

Arthrogryposis

Arthrogryposis is where a baby is born with mis-shapen joints. This condition is also known as arthrogryposis multiplex congenita.

It can affect many joints and mobility and dexterity can be affected. The muscles surrounding the joints may also be affected and might not form properly. Treatment is aimed at improving the function of the affected limbs with physiotherapy, splints and surgery. Occupational therapy can be important in allowing the child to interact with their surroundings as fully as possible. Children with conditions resulting in abnormal muscle or nerve development can also be born with this condition. Some affected children face mobility and self-care difficulties.

Children with arthrogryposis can be educated in mainstream and special schools. The extent to which this condition affects schooling depends on how movement has been limited and the medical interventions required. School-based *Interdisciplinary working* involving a physiotherapist and an occupational therapist will be necessary for most children while community medical services will manage others. Effective links with parents and good pastoral arrangements will be needed to provide children with support.

Children with arthrogryposis will need access to the same curriculum as their peers (see *Physical disability*). Special attention may be needed to gross and fine motor development, and it is not unusual to have to arrange for regular splinting and exercises to take place during the school day. Adaptations may be needed to aspects of the school environment – a good way of carrying out this work is to ask parents and the occupational therapist who knows the child to walk through the school. Scissors, pencils and pens and other standard learning implements may also need to be adapted. The advice of medical professionals might be needed to ensure that

exercises, activities and games in PE are appropriate.

Useful links
The Arthrogryposis Group (TAG)
1 The Oaks
Gillingham SP8 4SW
Tel/Fax: 01747 822655
E-mail: taguk@aol.com
http://tagonline.org.uk

Arthrogryposis multiplex congenita *see Arthrogryposis*

Artificial feeding

Artificial feeding is the term given to techniques for providing calories to children who are unable to chew, swallow or absorb food normally. This might be due to neurological problems that prevent normal eating and digestion, or other feeding problems. In some children a fine nasogastric tube is passed through a nostril and down the gullet into the stomach. Nutritious fluids can then be passed through the tube. The tube is stuck to the face with tape and is unsightly. This method is usually used for short periods of time. A more permanent way of accessing the stomach can be provided by surgically fashioning a hole between the abdominal wall and the stomach. This is called a gastrostomy. A gastrostomy tube can then be passed through the hole to provide feeds. These feeds can be given continuously, and may require a special pump, or can be given from time to time as discrete volumes of feed (bolus feeding). The gastrostomy is hidden under clothing and may therefore be better, cosmetically, for children. A gastrostomy can be used indefinitely and does not preclude normal feeding if this is possible or safe.

Children requiring artificial feeding can be educated in mainstream and special schools. Artificial feeding is more likely to affect children's schooling in the primary phase; older pupils will be more confident and independent. School-based *Interdisciplinary working* might be necessary for some children, while community medical services will manage others. Effective links with parents and good pastoral arrangements will provide support for these children.

Some children requiring artificial feeding will need special arrangements at break and lunch times – possibly a room that is not overly busy and is reasonably quiet. It is unlikely that the curriculum should be modified for these children.

Useful links
TOFS (Tracheo-Oesophageal Fistula Support)
St George's Centre
91 Victoria Road
Netherfield
Nottingham NG4 2NN
Tel: 0115 961 3092
E-mail: info@tofs.org.uk
www.tofs.org.uk
Some useful information sheets are available from this organisation.

Asperger's syndrome

Children with Asperger's syndrome will be more likely to have average or above aver-

age intelligence. As in autism and autistic spectrum disorders, it affects the child's ability to communicate, to interact with others and to use their imagination (see *Autism*).

Useful links
ACTION for ASD
Tel/Fax: 01706 222657
E-mail: info@actionasd.org.uk
www.actionasd.org.uk
ACTION for ASD is a registered charity, based in Lancashire UK. It is affiliated to the National Autistic Society.

National Autistic Society
393 City Road
London EC1 1NG
Tel: 020 7833 2299
E-mail: nas@nas.org.uk
www.oneworld.org/autism-uk

Asthma

Asthma is a common condition that affects as many as one in five school-aged children. It causes cough, wheeze and shortness of breath and can severely affect the child's ability to take part in sports and physical exercise. Treatment is mainly with inhalers that dilate the narrowed airways and/or prevent the airways narrowing in the first place. In many children, the asthma improves as they age. It is vital that all children with asthma have ready access to their 'reliever' inhalers (containing salbutamol [Ventolin] or terbutaline [Bricanyl]) to prevent severe attacks from becoming established. Asthma can coexist with *Eczema* and hay fever.

Children with asthma can be educated in mainstream and special schools. The extent to which asthma affects schooling depends on the medical interventions required. These conditions are usually managed simply by community medical services. Effective links with parents and good pastoral arrangements might be needed.

Children with asthma should not need any major adaptations to the curriculum, although it may be necessary to adjust the content of the PE curriculum to match what children can manage. Staff should be aware of the supportive things that they can do where there are allergies. Some families might want to explore diets excluding certain foods; schools can help parents by managing access to permitted foods and supervising snacks at break times and by observing children over time. Overall children with asthma have a condition that from time to time can interfere with their education.

Useful links
Action against Allergy
PO Box 278
Twickenham TW1 4QQ
Tel: 020 8892 2711
E-mail:
AAA@actionagainstallergy.freeserve.co.uk
www.actionagainstallergy.co.uk

Breathe Easy
British Lung Foundation
78 Hatton Garden
London EC1N 8LD
Tel: 020 7831 5831
E-mail: blf@britishlungfoundation.com
www.lunguk.org

British Allergy Foundation
Deepdene House
30 Bellegrove Road
Welling DA16 3PY
Tel: 020 8303 8583
E-mail: info@allergyfoundation.com
www.allergyfoundation.com

DfES Publications Centre
PO Box 5050
Sudbury CO10 6ZQ
Tel: 0845 602 2260
www.dfes.gov.uk/medical/

Supporting Pupils with Medical Needs – a Good Practice Guide *is a document for helping schools draw up policies on managing medication in schools, and to put in place effective management systems to support individual pupils with medical needs. This can be downloaded from the DfES Website.*

National Asthma Campaign
Providence House
Providence Place
London N1 0NT
Tel: 020 7226 2260

National Asthma Campaign Scotland
2a North Charlotte Street
Edinburgh EH2 4HR
Tel: 0131 226 2544
www.asthma.org.uk

National Society for Research into Allergies and Environmental Diseases
PO Box 45
Hinckley LE10 1JY
Tel/Fax: 01455 250715
E-mail: nsra.allergy@virgin.net

Ataxia

Ataxia means unsteadiness and can be due to a variety of causes. Cerebellar ataxia is unsteadiness due to a disorder affecting the part of the brain concerned with smoothing and coordinating movement. Other causes of ataxia can be due to illnesses affecting other parts of the brain or muscles. Drugs can also cause ataxia. Children taking the anticonvulsants carbamazepine or phenytoin might exhibit unsteadiness as a side effect. Older children and adolescents might exhibit (temporary) ataxia due to alcohol intoxication.

Children with ataxia can be educated in mainstream and special schools. School-based *Interdisciplinary working* involving a physiotherapist and an occupational therapist might be necessary for some children, while community medical services will manage others. Effective links with parents and good pastoral arrangements will provide support for these children.

Most difficulties are with mobility, fine motor activity and coordination. Attendant self-care difficulties can also occur. The advice about the school environment curriculum and resources found under *Physical disability* will apply.

Useful links
Friedreich's Ataxia Group
10 Winchester House
11 Cranmer Road
Kennington Park
London SW9 6EJ
Tel: 020 7820 3900
E-mail: office@ataxia.org.uk
www.ataxia.org.uk

Ataxic cerebral palsy *see* Cerebral palsy

Atrial septal defect (ASD)

ASD occurs when there is a hole between the collecting chambers of the heart. It rarely causes many symptoms unless the hole is very large, when breathlessness on exercise might be apparent. The flow of blood through the hole can increase the risk of infections of the heart (endocarditis). The treatment is surgical closure, although small holes can be closed off through a flexible tube (catheter). This condition can coexist with other heart defects.

For the child at school, the main impact of a large defect will be on their ability to take part in strenuous physical exercise (see *Congenital heart diseases*).

Atrioventricular septal defect

Atrioventricular septal defect occurs when the heart fails to form completely leaving a hole between the two sides of the heart that straddles both the collecting and the pumping chambers. The result is that abnormal amounts of blood flow back through the lungs. This causes breathlessness and growth difficulties in babies. The condition is seen in babies born with *Down's syndrome*. Operative treatment is required to address the problem. This condition can coexist with other heart defects (see *Congenital heart diseases*).

Attention deficit disorder (ADD) see Attention deficit hyperactivity disorder (ADHD)

Attention deficit hyperactivity disorder (ADHD)

Children with ADHD have various combinations of impairment in perception, conceptualisation, language, memory, control of attention, impulse and motor function. The core difficulties are those of inattentiveness, distractibility and motor restlessness. The term attention deficit disorder (ADD) refers to the condition when there are no symptoms of motor restlessness. A further defining factor is the absence of other significant learning difficulties, although there is overlap between ADHD, developmental coordination disorder (*Dyspraxia*) and *Dyslexia*. The child's difficulties may be further compounded by behavioural difficulties that might arise as a result of the ADHD.

School-based *Interdisciplinary working,* including the advice of an educational psychologist, who has specialised in this work, and a specialist teacher, is desirable. Effective links with parents can be very helpful. Good pastoral arrangements will provide support for these children and include opportunities to celebrate success and reinforce self-esteem. Children on stimulant medication (methylphenidate) as part of the multimodal treatment programme for the condition will require monitoring at home and school. Good communication between the two is vital to ensure that all strategies put in place to help the child learn complement one another.

It is very important to ensure that all staff are appropriately informed through training of how ADHD affects educational attainment. Children with ADHD can easily attract negative responses and these can lead to unnecessarily low expectations and to a climate of failure. It is vital to develop a whole school perspective that will reinforce the positive aspects of these children. In particular, staff must strive to respond positively to children who, because of their condition, may show little attention to detail and make careless mistakes, might not listen when spoken to directly, might not follow instructions and are easily distracted. They may forget things or forget instructions. They may fidget, leave their seat in the classroom, run about or climb excessively at inappropriate times. They might have difficulty playing quietly and can talk excessively. Their impulsivity can lead to blurting out answers before questions are completed, difficulty awaiting their turn and interrupting or intruding on others. Any of these can be the source of disruption to lessons and to the learning of a whole class.

In school, children with ADHD can be helped by giving attention to the learning environment, communication, teaching strategies and the management of behaviour. The advice of parents is generally useful before starting the planning of an educational programme. Where a child is starting a new school, arrange an orientation or induction visit with parents. The individual education plan needs to be specific and detailed. For some children it might be important to establish dietary requirements and to ensure that inappropriate foods are not easily available. In the classroom make sure that pupils with ADHD sit near the teacher's desk towards the front with their backs to the rest of the class to keep distractions to a minimum. Try not to place students with ADHD near heaters, or doors or windows or any other distracting stimuli or source of noise. If possible create a stimuli-reduced study area, such as a workstation – make this accessible to all pupils, but use it for the child with ADHD when it is required. Take care with the management of change, as new schedules and unplanned events can lead to heightened disruption.

In order to communicate well with children with ADHD, it is important to develop the skills of all staff. They will need to maintain eye contact during verbal instruction, make directions clear and concise and be consistent with regularly used daily instructions. Multiple commands should be avoided and complex directions simplified; if needed, instructions should be repeated in a calm and positive manner. Check that children understand instructions before beginning a task or activity. For wider communication it might be useful to establish a daily notebook or diary, as this can be used to note work covered in school and to confirm homework. This also serves as a means of communicating between home and school.

Effective teaching strategies for children with ADHD are generally good teaching methods for all children. Make sure that the lesson has an obvious and clear structure with a beginning, middle and end. Tell students in advance what they will learn, provide good resources, give written as well as oral instructions, summarise and check on what has been learnt. In lessons it is a good idea to give children with ADHD one task at a time, monitoring progress frequently. Give extra time for certain tasks, as children with ADHD tend to work slowly. Ensure that short-term plans are suitably differentiated to take account of particular needs and make the best of specific strengths. Children with ADHD are easily frustrated. Stress, pressure and fatigue can break down their self-control, leading to disruptive behaviour: in these situations support staff are invaluable in monitoring and identifying signs and symptoms of stress in sufficient time to manage the situation.

It is very important for the school to have good behaviour management policy and practices that are consistently used and applied by all staff. Keep school and class rules to a minimum and keep them simple; try to express rules as those things children should do rather than telling them what they should not. Avoid debating or arguing about misconduct, move swiftly to consequences and do not criticise, as some children with ADHD find it very difficult to maintain self-control. Always note good things and praise appropriate behaviour and performance. Take time to find those things that motivate and use these as rewards. Build and develop high esteem in every possible situation and whenever possible get the child to recognise their own success.

Useful links
ADD/ADHD Family Support Group
1a High Street
Dilton Marsh
Westbury BA13 4DL
Tel: 01373 826045

ADDiss Information Services
PO Box 340
Edgware HA8 9HL
Tel: 020 8906 9068
E-mail: books@addiss.co.uk
www.addiss.co.uk

The ADHD National Alliance
209–211 City Road
London EC1V 1JN
Tel: 020 7608 8760
E-mail: jim@cafamily.org.uk

The Henry Spink Foundation
209–211 City Road
London EC1V 1JN
Tel: 020 7608 8789
E-mail: info@henryspink.org
www.henryspink.org

Hyperactive Children's Support Group
71 Whyke Lane
Chichester PO19 2LD
Tel: 01243 551313
E-mail: hacsg@hacsg.org.uk
www.hacsg.org.uk

NARA (National Action & Research for
ADHD)
Glenrosa, Lightlands Lane
Cookham SL6 9DH
Tel: 01628 523539
E-mail: AngieT8282@aol.com

Parentline Plus
Endway House
Hadleigh SS7 2AN
Tel: 0808 800 2222
E-mail: helpline@parentlineplus.org. uk
www.parentline.co.uk

Auditory agnosia

Auditory agnosia is the inability of the brain to make sense or interpret sounds heard by the child. It can occur in certain types of epilepsy, where the parts of the brain concerned with understanding sounds are affected (see *Laundau–Kleffner syndrome*).

Children with auditory agnosia are, or become, unable to interpret speech or assign meaning to the sounds that they hear. This limits speech and communication and has a significant impact on learning. Hearing tests can show normal hearing. Some children for no apparent reason begin to have trouble understanding what is said to them. Where this happens doctors and other professionals find well-documented classroom-based language development records invaluable. It is not unusual for parents to think that their child is developing a hearing problem or has become suddenly deaf.

Children with auditory agnosia can be educated in mainstream and special schools. School-based *Interdisciplinary working* involving specialist teachers and speech and language therapists might be necessary for some children, while community medical services will manage others. Effective links with parents and good pastoral arrangements will provide support for these children.

The complexities of working with children with auditory agnosia will be determined by the extent to which understanding is lost. The inability to understand language eventually affects the child's spoken language, which can progress to a complete loss of the ability to speak (*Mutism*). Children who have learned to read and write before the onset of auditory agnosia can often continue communicating through written language. Some children are capable of communication using a sign language. The child's intelligence usually appears unaffected; however, because of frustration and communication problems, there may be behavioural or psychological problems. Work with peers will be necessary so that they understand the condition and do not overreact to situations or exacerbate communication frustration. A withdrawal room can be useful, as it will minimise interruptions to lessons.

Autism

Autism is a condition where development of communication, social interaction and cognition are affected. Children often present with delayed or absent speech, limited interaction with other members of their family (for example, poor eye contact) and restricted or repetitive behaviours (for instance, spinning objects or lining up toys in the same way). Learning difficulties are often severe and affected children are more prone to *Epilepsy*. Where learning difficulty is less marked and speech develops, the child is said to have high functioning autism or *Asperger syndrome*.

Children with autism find it hard or impossible to make sense of the world because of their difficulties with social relatedness and other learning difficulties, and they require a great deal of understanding from all those working with them. Children with autism can have a wide range of abilities affected variously in the domains of social communication, social interaction and imag-

ination; this is often referred to as the triad of impairments. Some children will have severe learning disabilities and require highly specialised educational provision; some will manage in mainstream with support, and others will be able to access the education system with minimal support.

It is very important for staff working with pupils with autism to have training and to develop an understanding of the condition. Teachers and support staff are going to be more effective if they have some understanding of what it is like to live in a world that is literal, to be without social intuition and to be very limited in imagination. Staff should be highly adaptable, creative and willing to tirelessly explore the many avenues of communication in search of the 'best fit'.

Children with autism benefit from order, as they like predictability in all aspects of their lives. Their education could include:

- a communication system that has been individually designed
- a means or system whereby activities and tasks can be worked through in a systematic way
- access to uncluttered quiet spaces
- access to spaces where energy can be released
- the need to develop good self-help and independence skills
- a carefully designed social skills programme
- a leisure skills programme including the capacity to make suitable things happen at times when things are not organised.

Considerable thought and attention needs to be given to the ways that teaching and learning is organised for the child. The environment needs to be predictable, unfussy and uncluttered. Changes and the extent to which changes can be handled by the child will vary; parents will often provide useful insights. Furniture and position can be important; it is not unusual for particular patterns or settings to be more acceptable than others. The management of time has to be considered – the way we describe time and the passage of time is abstract, so it is useful to find a concrete means of communicating the passage of time. This will help with the anticipation of change and therefore provide the child with greater understanding. It is good to get a means of indicating the start of something, a day, a lesson, a break, and then finding a way of showing how long it will take the unit of time to pass and finally to mark the end. During the school day, children will need help with organising themselves – picture timetables and picture templates can be very helpful.

Forms of communication for children with autism might be highly individualised, in which case it will be important to have the advice of a speech and language therapist and/or a specialist teacher (see *Interdisciplinary working*). It is beyond the scope of this section to give details of the many communication programmes that can be used. Generally, communication should be adapted and make best use of those methods the child is already using. Because children with autism use and interpret speech literally, it is sensible to avoid idioms, colloquialisms, double meanings, sarcasm, jokes and nicknames; it is better to be as concrete as possible using short and clear sentences. Within as consistent and

predictable an environment as possible, children may need to learn to use objects, pictures, symbols, written words, sounds, signs or spoken words. Because children with autism are likely to have difficulty with abstract information, it is helpful to use a medium that is likely to appeal to their visual and spatial skills. The Picture Exchange Communication System (PECS) is used in many special schools and proves a good and dependable way of initiating and developing a child's capacity to communicate. Parents will know their children best and can be very helpful, particularly when a communication programme is being designed.

The rigidity of some children can lead them to be distressed when the unpredictable happens. It is useful to establish a 'safe place' or identify a 'safe person' as part of a strategy of support. It is important to develop a consistent whole-school approach to supporting the child's capacity to deal with unplanned changes.

Teachers and staff inexperienced in working with children and young people with autistic spectrum disorders will need to get good advice; most education departments will have suitable information and specialist outreach teams.

A number of special treatments or educational interventions are available worldwide. These have attracted considerable publicity and recent interest from the media including:

- Daily Life Therapy (Higashi)
- 'TEACCH' (Treatment and Education of Autistic Children and related Communication Handicaps [sic])
- 'Options' (an interactive approach developed in the USA)

- Irlen (the use of coloured lenses in spectacles to address perceptual difficulties)
- Special diets
- Tomatis approach (auditory integration)
- Secretin injections
- Lovaas (intensive interaction based on a behavioural approach)
- SPELL (Structure, Positive approaches, Empathy, Low arousal, Links with parents) – an approach developed by the National Autistic Society designed to address the triad of impairments)
- Earlybird (a National Autistic Society preschool project originating in Barnsley)
- PECS (Picture Exchange Communication System)
- a variety of musical interactive approaches, etc.

The recent interest and requests by parents for one or more approaches to be available led to a review for the DfES (for details, see below). This provides interesting reading. Many schools and units will successfully use one or more specialist strategies and programmes and adapt them according to their circumstances.

Some children with autism will demonstrate frustration and challenging behaviours in certain situations – it is important that adults working with these children are carefully trained in strategies for low arousal and, where necessary, in safe and positive handling.

Overall children with autism have a condition that will impact on their education and this requires modifications to the delivery and content of the curriculum.

Useful links
DfES Publications Centre
PO Box 5050
Sudbury CO10 6ZQ
Tel: 0845 602 2260
www.dfes.gov.uk/medical/

Jordan R., Jones G., Mamight D. Educational Interventions for Children with Autism: a Literature Review of Recent and Current Research. Sudbury: DfEE, 1998. ISBN 0 85 5228538 5 £4.95.

National Autistic Society
393 City Road
London EC1 1NG
Tel: 020 7833 2299
E-mail: nas@nas.org.uk
www.oneworld.org/autism-uk

Society For The Autistically Handicapped (SFTH)
199–205 Blandford Avenue
Kettering NN16 9AT
Tel: 01536 523274
E-mail: autism@rmplc.co.uk
www.rmplc.co.uk/eduweb/sites/autism/
www.autismconnect.org
Site organised with support of NAS that aims to be the first port of call for anyone interested in autism, providing news, events, world maps and rapid access to other websites with information on autism.

B

Battarism

Battarism causes increasingly clumsy and rapid speech after involuntary repetition or mistakes of pronunciation (see *Speech disorder*).

Becker muscular dystrophy *see* Duchenne muscular dystrophy

Bed wetting *see* Neuropathic bladder; Nocturnal enuresis

Birthmarks *see* Strawberry naevus

Blindness

Most children who are registered blind have some residual vision and are able to use a significant amount of their remaining visual function – see *Visual impairment*. A number of registered blind children have no vision and will need highly specialised programmes based on developing their other senses including touch, hearing and smell. A very small number of children are deaf and blind – see *Deafblind*. It is important for blind children to be trained to develop their other senses in ways that will give them the greatest access to the world and to learning. Because such training is highly specialised, it is beyond the scope of this entry to provide more than a general outline of those elements of schooling that need specific attention.

Some children who are blind can be educated in mainstream schools, while others will need highly specialised environments with trained and skilled staff in special units or in special schools. Attention should be given to the child, the environment and curriculum. School-based *Interdisciplinary working* will be necessary, including the regular attention and advice of a specialist teacher for visually impaired children. The earliest possible intervention through paediatric clinics and preschool services is necessary. Effective links with parents and good pastoral arrangements will provide support for these children.

The monitoring of a pupil's well-being during the school day is vital, as fatigue and anxiety may affect their abilities to engage with their world and their work. In all planning it is important to build in sufficient time for a pupil to do whatever is required – for example, a pupil reading by touch will need more time allowed for work to be completed. Mobility arrangements will be individually determined with advice from a mobility specialist and/or the advice of a specialist teacher of the visually impaired. A mobility plan will be a vital element of a pupil's programme; this will need maintaining and extending as the pupil progresses. Careful planning is needed to prepare children for changes or new environments, for example at times of transition or school trips. Hooples, canes and sticks are made for all kinds of needs and they include lightweight and fold-away versions. Guide dogs are not usually available until after the age of 16.

The school environment will not need the kind of attention required for visually impaired children, such as colour and contrast; however, there are many useful sensory adaptations and additions that can easily be put into place to support the blind child. It is sensible to ask the specialist teacher of the visually impaired and the mobility officer/specialist to audit the school site and provide a list of modifications. It is useful to know which are essential and which are desirable.

To support curriculum access, information using recorded media will be required. There is a wide range of recorded material for the cassette and compact disc player. Cassette and compact disc players are widely available in schools. It is very important to develop the use of recorded media as this will provide a lifetime access to information. A vast range of 'Talking Books, Magazines and Newspapers' is available for purchase or loan from local groups and outlets. Access to the world of information is easily available through the Internet and the technology of turning screen-based information into audio is rapidly developing; similarly, the rapid development of voice-activated software provides the means of producing text. Advice and possibly a communication assessment should be sought including applications of technology to support learning.

Reading text by touch is a skill requiring specialised teaching. The two systems most often used are Braille and Moon. Braille letters are formed with different combinations of six dots; Moon letters are based on the shapes of conventionally printed letters and therefore ideal for those that have knowledge of print. Standardised assessment tests (SATs) will be needed in Braille, and there is useful advice on this on the Royal National Institute for the Blind's www.rnib.org.uk/curriculum/exams.htm site.

It can be very helpful to develop the role of sighted peers by encouraging them to be aware of the implications of the blindness of their classmate. Sighted peers can greatly assist by encouraging and supporting. Care needs to be taken over arrangements of this kind, as the independence and confidence of a blind pupil is important.

Useful links
Hands and Eyes
A USA specialist teacher maintains this useful online newsletter for teachers and caregivers of visually impaired students and their friends. It includes art, cooking and manipulative activities that visually impaired students can do individually or in small groups. It is for teachers and support staff in need of ideas for classroom activities and is particularly useful for pupils with multiple impairments such as developmental disability and motor impairment.
www.home.earthlink.net/~vharris/

RNIB Education Information Services
224 Great Portland Street
London W1N 6AA
Tel: 020 7388 1266
E-mail: webmaster@rnib.org.uk
www.rnib.org.uk
RNIB's curriculum information service offers information and advice to all professionals supporting a visually impaired child in mainstream or special schools.
www.rnib.org.uk/curriculum/
RNIB's accessing technology pages provide information about applications of technology in employment, at study and in leisure.
www.rnib.org.uk/technology/

V.I. Guide
This site contains information on many topics relat-

ing to parenting and teaching a child with visual impairments.

www.viguide.com/

Bow legs

Bow legs are when the legs appear to bow outwards and are usually most noticeable in young children when they first start walking. They normally straighten gradually on their own. In some children the legs are bowed because of vitamin D deficiency (*Rickets*) but this is now fortunately quite rare.

Useful links
STEPS
Lymm Court
11 Eagle Brow
Lymm WA13 0LP
Tel: 01925 757525
E-mail: info@steps-charity.org.uk
www.steps-charity.org.uk

Brain haemorrhage

Brain haemorrhage can occur in children and can produce effects similar to that of a stroke in an adult. It can be caused by the bleeding of abnormal blood vessels in the brain or abnormal clotting of the blood. This means the child might be left with permanent mobility, speech, visual or cognitive problems.

Children who have had strokes can be educated in mainstream and special schools. Some children will recover well from strokes and not require additional help, while others may experience a range of mild to severe consequences including a range of educa-

tional implications (see *Hearing impairment, Visual impairment, Head injury, Epilepsy* and *Cerebral palsy*). School-based *Interdisciplinary working* involving therapists and specialist workers might be necessary for some children, although others will have their condition managed by community medical services. Effective links with parents and good pastoral arrangements will provide support for these children. Overall children with brain haemorrhage or strokes have a variable condition that is likely to affect their education.

Useful links
Different Strokes
162 High Street
Watford WD1 2EG
Tel: 01923 240615
E-mail: info@differentstrokes.co.uk
www.differentstrokes.co.uk

Brain tumours

Brain tumours cause symptoms owing to the direct effect of the tumour on the affected part of the brain, and also by increasing the pressure within the skull. Children may present with headache, nausea, vomiting or with visual problems. They can also develop weaknesses, *Epilepsy* or unsteadiness in walking. Some children undergo personality or behavioural changes or experience learning difficulty. Treatment can be with surgery, radiotherapy or with drugs (chemotherapy). Some treatments can result in residual impairments for the child.

Children with brain tumours can be educated in mainstream and special schools. Brain tumours will have some effect on education, as complex medical interventions usually requiring hospitalisation are required. When children are in hospital, effective liaison with the hospital education service will help maintain the curriculum and learning. School-based *Interdisciplinary working* may be necessary for some children, while community medical services will manage others. Effective links with parents and good pastoral arrangements will provide support for these children in all aspects of their school life.

Frequent absence from school and time-consuming treatments might be required – these can lead to staff having low expectations and can disrupt school friendships. It is important to explore all possible ways of supporting children who are regularly absent and to provide a range of ways to help them catch up with work; this becomes very important where children are mid-syllabus for externally accredited examinations. Sometimes, children with brain tumours will experience side effects from their treatment – for example they may regress and lose physical skills, communication skills, general cognitive abilities, and senses might be affected; children can change in attitude and personality and become depressed. In these situations schools will need to provide considerable support to child and family. A highly differentiated curriculum will need additional support and advice from specialist teachers.

Useful links
Brain Tumour Foundation
PO Box 162
New Malden KT3 4WH
Tel/Fax: 020 8336 2020
E-mail: btf.uk@virgin.net

Brittle bone disease

Brittle bone disease is a rare disease where the bones do not form normally and are prone to break. The condition is called osteogenesis imperfecta. Affected children might suffer from multiple fractures that occur from birth onwards during normal day-to-day activities. The bones are often deformed and lack calcium. Children can have severe pain and limb or joint deformity with consequent mobility and handling problems. The bones, once fractured, do not heal well.

Treatment can be with orthopaedic surgery and some children will need appropriate aids and appliances, for instance a powered wheelchair. Recently, drugs have been made available that increase the strength of the bone and reduce the number of fractures.

Children with brittle bone disease can be educated in mainstream and special schools. The extent to which this condition affects schooling depends on the medical interventions required. Some children will experience a number of long periods of restricted mobility and will need exercises designed by a physiotherapist. School-based *Interdisciplinary working* involving a physiotherapist and an occupational therapist might be necessary for some children, while community medical services will manage others. Effective links with parents and good pastoral arrangements will provide support for these children.

Children with brittle bone disease will need access to the same curriculum as their peers. Frequent absence from school and time-consuming treatments can lead to low expectations. It is important to explore all possible ways of supporting children who are regularly absent and to provide a range of ways to help them catch up with work, particularly where children are mid-syllabus for externally accredited examinations. Some children will spend long periods in wheelchairs and therefore access to classrooms and buildings needs to be good. Detailed work requiring fine motor skills should be adapted; some children cannot hold pencils easily and may need specialised keyboard access. The advice of medical professionals might be needed to ensure that exercises, activities and games in PE are appropriate.

Useful links
Brittle Bone Society
30 Guthrie Street
Dundee DD1 5BS
Tel: 08000 282459
E-mail: bbs@brittlebone.org
www.brittlebone.org

Bronchiectasis

Bronchiectasis is a condition where parts of the lungs become damaged by infections and thereafter act as an ongoing source of further infection and damage. Children with this condition often have a cough and bring up phlegm. They might need frequent courses of antibiotics (by mouth or even intravenously) and physiotherapy to help get rid of the lung secretions.

Children with bronchiectasis can be educated in mainstream and special schools. This condition is usually managed by community medical services. School-based *Interdisciplinary working* will be necessary

including the regular attention and advice of a physiotherapist. Effective links with parents and good pastoral arrangements will be needed to give children support.

Children with bronchiectasis will need access to the same curriculum as their peers. Staff will need to have high expectations and be aware of the things that will be needed to support children and keep them healthy. Some children will have severe coughing attacks, occasionally coughing up mucus, and the physical management of this is important. Physiotherapy sessions should be built into the school day with the minimum disruption to the curriculum; it may be possible for these to take place at break times. A separate room or area will be needed for chest physiotherapy. Special consideration should be given to sporting activities. Although PE is beneficial, some children seem lethargic following illness. Overall children with bronchiectasis have a condition that will occasionally interfere with their education.

Useful links
Breathe Easy
British Lung Foundation
78 Hatton Garden
London EC1N 8LD
Tel: 020 7831 5831
E-mail: blf@britishlungfoundation.com
www.lunguk.org

Bullying

Bullying can be a source of considerable distress and anxiety for many children. All schools are legally required under the School

Standards and Framework Act 1998 to draw up procedures to prevent bullying among pupils and to bring these procedures to the attention of staff, parents and pupils. It is very important that all staff promote a culture and ethos within which bullying is not accepted. The school's pastoral system should provide support to the child being bullied. Children who bully need to be worked with to help them to manage their aggression and to be taught social responsibility.

The significance of bullying is often underestimated. Research shows that at least 40 per cent of children experience some kind of bullying during their school career and that this adversely affects their work and emotional well-being.

Those schools that have good pastoral procedures/practices, good behaviour management, supervise pupils well, and have clear action where discipline is required and where pupils understand that responsibility for behaviour extends beyond the site and the school day are less likely to have problems with bullying.

Useful links
Bullying Online
www.bullying.co.uk
www.dfes.gov.uk/bullying/
This website is intended to show pupils, their families and teachers how to tackle the problem of bullying.

Bophthalmos *see* Glaucome

Burns

Burns cause scarring and disfigurement, depending on the site and severity of the injury. For severe burns, much time from school can be lost.

Children who have had burns can be educated in schools and during some treatments in hospital schools. The extent to which the consequences of burns and their treatment affect schooling depends on the severity of the injuries and the extent of the medical interventions required. For some children pain management is important; others may experience long periods of restricted mobility and will need exercises designed by a physiotherapist. School-based *Interdisciplinary working* might be necessary for some children, while community medical services will manage others. Effective links with parents and good pastoral arrangements will provide support for these children.

At times some children can appear very different because of skin grafts; classmates should be encouraged to be supportive to avoid any unnecessary comments (see *Disfigurement and difference*).

Children who have had burns will need access to the same curriculum as their peers. They can present as underachievers because of their frequent absence from school and they have lower expectations because of the effects of their burns. Some children will require treatment during the day – this is usually possible outside class teaching time. A school needs good systems of support and opportunities for children to catch up after absences following treatments. Children in the primary phase may need special attention; they might not tell staff when there is discomfort or a problem with a dressing, because they are engrossed in a particular activity or because they might prefer to avoid treatment. Special arrangements will probably be needed to provide access to some sporting activities.

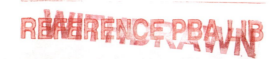

Useful links
British Association of Dermatologists
19 Fitzroy Square
London W1T 6EH
Tel: 020 7383 0266
Fax: 020 7388 5263
E-mail: admin@bad.org.uk
www.skinhealth.co.uk/contact/index.htm

Burns Support Group
www.burnsupportgroupsdatabase.com/

C

Café au lait patches *see* Neurofibromatosis

Cancer

Cancer is an umbrella term that refers to a group of conditions where parts of the body grow without the normal controlling mechanisms that limit growth and multiplication of the cells. The cells can overgrow in a particular area causing a lump (or tumour), and also invade or spread to surrounding or distant parts of the body (see under specific entries, for instance *Brain tumours, Leukaemia, Lymphoma, Osteosarcoma, Retinoblastoma* and *Wilms tumour*).

Treatment often has an impact on the emotional and psychological well-being of the child and family.

Children with cancers can be educated in mainstream, special and hospital schools. School-based *Interdisciplinary working* might be necessary for some children, while many will have their condition managed by hospital and community medical services. Effective links with parents and good pastoral arrangements will provide support for these children. Cancer may mean some children experience long and frequent periods of illness together with complex courses of treatment. Frequent absence from school for time-consuming treatments can lead to staff having low expectations of children's achievements and to school friendships being disrupted. It is important to explore all possible ways of supporting children who are regularly absent and to provide a range of ways to help them catch up with work; this becomes very important where children are mid-syllabus for externally accredited examinations. Side effects of cancer treatment need sensitive management. Children with cancer will need access to the same curriculum as their peers.

Useful links
CancerBACUP
3 Bath Place
Rivington Street
London EC2A 3JR
Tel: 020 7696 9003
E-mail: info@cancerbacup.org
www.cancerbacup.org.uk

Cancer Care Society
11 The Cornmarket
Romsey SO51 8GB
Tel: 01794 830300

Cancerlink
Macmillan Cancer Relief
89 Albert Embankment
London SE1 7UQ
Tel: 0808 808 0000/020 7840 7840
E-mail: cancerlink@cancerlink.org.uk
www.cancerlink.org

CLIC
Abbey Wood
Bristol BS34 7JU
Tel: 0117 311 2600
E-mail: clic@charity.demon.co.uk
www.clic.uk.com

Edward's Trust
Edward House

St Mary's Row
Birmingham B4 6NY
Tel: 0121 237 5656

Cardiomyopathies

Cardiomyopathies are conditions where the muscle of the heart is damaged, sometimes following virus infections. Treatment is with drugs to minimise the strain on the heart and, in some children, heart transplantation is required.

Children with these problems may find it hard to take part in physical exercise (see *Congenital heart diseases*).

Cataract

A cataract is an opacity in the normally clear lens of the eye. It can be due to a variety of conditions, for instance *Mucopolysaccharidosis* or *Down's syndrome*. Some children are born with the condition (congenital cataracts) while, in other babies, infection in the womb during development causes the cataract (for example, rubella). The cataract can range from small and insignificant through to opacities severe enough to produce severe visual handicap. Treatment involves the surgical removal of the cataract, which can then often be replaced by an artificial implantable lens.

Children with cataracts can be educated in mainstream and special schools. They will need care and attention before and during removal of the cataract. School-based *Interdisciplinary working* might be necessary for some children, while others will have their condition simply managed based on community medical services. Curriculum implications are usually minimal and largely depend on the extent to which treatment affects vision. Before a cataract is removed a child is likely to experience some difficulties including double or multiple vision, difficulties with colours and poor night vision. Special spectacles are usually prescribed to correct vision; the eye is likely to be rather sensitive to bright light.

Useful links
Hands and Eyes
A USA specialist teacher maintains this useful online newsletter for teachers and caregivers of visually impaired students and their friends. It includes art, cooking and manipulative activities that visually impaired students can do individually or in small groups. It is for teachers and support staff in need of ideas for classroom activities and is particularly useful for pupils with multiple impairments such as developmental disability and motor impairment.
www.home.earthlink.net/~vharris/

RNIB Education Information Services
224 Great Portland Street
London W1N 6AA
Tel: 020 7388 1266
E-mail: webmaster@rnib.org.uk
www.rnib.org.uk
RNIB's curriculum information service offers information and advice to all professionals supporting a visually impaired child in mainstream or special schools.
www.rnib.org.uk/curriculum/
RNIB's accessing technology pages provide information about applications of technology in employment, at study and in leisure.
www.rnib.org.uk/technology/

V.I. Guide
This site contains information on many topics relating to parenting and teaching a child with visual impairments.
www.viguide.com/

Cerebellar ataxia *see* Ataxia

Cerebral palsy

Cerebral palsy most noticeably affects movement because of damage to the developing brain during pregnancy, birth and early on in childhood. Although the damage to the brain does not worsen as the child grows, the corresponding elongation and growth of the bones, joints and muscles mean that the effects on movement might change. The muscles are usually stiffer than normal (spasticity or hypertonia) and weaker (paretic or plegic). Various parts of the body can be affected. Where just one limb is affected, the child is said to have a monoplegia. When one half of the body is affected, it is called hemiplegia. Where the legs are predominantly affected then this is called diplegia. When all four limbs are affected the child has paraplegia also known as tetraplegia or four-limb cerebral palsy. It can also make muscles weaker than normal and the control mechanisms can be damaged leading to unsteadiness (ataxic cerebral palsy). In some the condition produces unwanted movements (dystonic cerebral palsy, choreoathetosis). Cerebral palsy can also affect the vision, ability to talk, chew and swallow, digestion and continence. Because the condition is caused by damage to the developing brain, there is an increased risk of epilepsy in affected children. Although some children

with cerebral palsy have severe learning difficulties, many have normal learning ability despite their physical difficulties.

Although children may encounter a wide range of physical, perceptual, intellectual, nutritional and continence difficulties, which threaten their potential for learning and independence, many needs can be met by timely input from physiotherapy, occupational therapy, speech and language therapy and medical, surgical and orthopaedic specialists (see *Interdisciplinary working*).

Children with cerebral palsy will be educated in all types of schools depending on needs and the organisation of schools locally. The advice found under *Physical disability* will apply. An individual educational programme should be designed to include developing movement skills, expressive and receptive communication, access to a suitably differentiated broad and balanced curriculum, self-help and independence skills, and social and daily living skills.

Children with cerebral palsy will need to overcome the barriers and constraints imposed by everyday life. It is important for teachers and parents to foster in children a determination to achieve their goals. For some children with cerebral palsy the emphasis on small group work, body awareness, concentration and problem solving found under *Conductive education* are known to be beneficial.

Useful links
HemiHelp
Bedford House
215 Balham High Road
London SW17 7BQ
Tel: 020 8672 3179
www.hemihelp.org.uk

Scope
6 Market Road
London N7 9PW
Tel:0808 800 3333
E-mail: cphelpline@scope.org.uk
www.scope.org.uk

CHARGE association

This is a rare set of congenital difficulties owing to loss of genetic material from chromosome 22. Babies born with the condition usually have heart defects, weakness of some of the facial muscles, *Coloboma*, underdevelopment of the nasal passages leading to blockage, difficulties with feeding, swallowing and gaining weight. They can also have deafness, malformations of the ear, abnormally formed genitals, low muscle tone and delayed development with later learning difficulties.

Children with CHARGE association can be educated in mainstream and special schools. Good pastoral support arrangements and school-based *Interdisciplinary working* will be important. It is important to have effective liaison and communication with parents and carers. Many children will have complex needs depending on which aspects of the association predominate; they will require a highly specialised environment and curriculum and high levels of additional support throughout the school day.

Useful links
CHARGE Association
82 Gwendoline Avenue
Upton Park
London E13 0RD

Tel: 020 8552 6961
E-mail: levey2000@cs.com
www.sense.org.uk/sensory_impairment/ch arge.html

Child abuse

Child abuse can affect any child at any time. The abuse can be physical, sexual, emotional or in the form of neglect. While physical abuse might sometimes be obvious, the other forms of abuse still cause distress in the child and can lead to signs and symptoms that can show themselves at school. Physical abuse might take the form of smacking, hitting, punching, pinching, biting, kicking or burning. Children can also be hit with implements such as belts or shoes. Burns, bruises, fractures and other (sometimes serious or life-threatening) injuries may result. Sexual abuse can range from exposing a child to pornography, inappropriate touching or fondling, through to rape, buggery or other indecent sexual assault. Children might disclose incidents of sexual abuse to teachers or might behave in an inappropriately sexualised manner. While emotional abuse can be harder to define, it still causes many problems for the child including school failure, growth failure, withdrawal from normal functioning/learning in school or emotional and behavioural problems.

All professionals working with children have a duty of care to inform the appropriate authorities if they suspect the child might have been, or is at significant risk of abuse. Where it is known that children have been abused the active involvement of professionals from other supporting agencies may be required (see *Interdisciplinary working*). Curriculum access and classroom performance can suffer significantly. Care should be given to the balance between confidentiality about pupils' circumstances and some staff needing to be aware of signs and indications of abuse in those pupils. All staff need to be well trained and pastoral systems need to be efficient and effective in order to ensure that children are protected. In circumstances where children are known to have experienced trauma through abuse, teachers might need to modify curriculum content to avoid painful reminders.

Good child protection procedures and policies are vital in all schools. It is essential that they are given a high priority in the school's selection and induction of new staff and are regularly reviewed. The local Area Child Protection Committee (ACPC) advises on and reviews local practice and procedure for inter-agency cooperation and training with regard to children in need of protection by local authorities. It is made up of representatives from various professions and agencies concerned with children. Schools must follow the advice given by their local ACPC.

Useful links
British Association for the Study and Prevention of Child Abuse and Neglect
10 Priory Street
York YO1 6EZ
Tel: 01904 613605
E-mail: baspcan@baspcan.org.uk
www.baspcan.org.uk

The National Association for People Abused in Childhood

Union House
Shepherds Bush Green
London W12 8UA
Tel: 020 8735 5009
E-mail: info@napac.org.uk
www.napac.org.uk

National Society for the Prevention of Cruelty to Children (NSPCC)
Weston House
42 Curtain Road
London EC2A 3NH
Tel: 020 7825 2500
www.nspcc.org.uk/html/homepage/home.htm

Choreoathetosis *see* Cerebral palsy

Chronic ambulatory peritoneal dialysis *see* Renal dialysis

Chronic fatigue syndrome

Chronic fatigue syndrome or myalgic encephalomyelitis (ME) causes excessive fatigue or tiredness. It can occur following a 'flu-like illness and has also been called postviral fatigue syndrome. The fatigue is both physical and mental. In some children the symptoms can be the result of a depressive illness, while in others the fatigue itself can lead to emotional and mood problems. The symptoms can be long lasting and can range from mild fatigability that does little to impede access to the normal school curriculum, through to very severe physical restriction that results in the child being confined to bed. The social isolation caused by the condition cannot be overstated.

Treatments are still developing, but a graded programme of gentle rehabilitation seems to be practically useful and effective for most sufferers. Psychological techniques, such as cognitive behavioural therapy, have also been used successfully in some cases.

Children who experience significant fatigue will need support and flexibility in order to give them the best possible access to all that the school provides. It is necessary to work closely with family and the wider multidisciplinary team (see *Interdisciplinary working*). If possible it is useful to provide a discreet place for rest and, if necessary, somewhere to sleep. In extreme circumstances, it is necessary to reconfigure the curriculum and identify core subjects that the child can attempt. It is particularly useful to know and work through the child's interests and hobbies. Some children require home tuition for periods of time.

Useful links
Association of Young People with ME
PO Box 605
Milton Keynes MK2 2XD
Tel: 01908 373300
E-mail: info@ayme.org.uk
www.ayme.org.uk

The National Association for the Education of Sick Children, NAESC, provides full-time education through the Satellite School with curriculum for the chronically sick (including those who have ME/CFS), pupils recovering from illness/injury, special needs, school-phobics, excluded pupils, and children whose parents prefer home education.

The Satellite School
Regus House
Herald Way
Pegasus Business Park
Castle Donington DE74 2TZ
Tel: 01332 638599
E-mail: satelliteschool@aol.com
www.satelliteschool.org.uk

Circumcision

Circumcision is the surgical removal of the foreskin from the end (glans) of the penis. It might be performed for religious reasons or as treatment for a tight foreskin that prevents urine from being passed easily (phimosis). The curriculum will not need to be modified for boys because they have been circumcised.

Cleft lip and palate

Cleft lip and palate can occur as congenital problems independently of one another or together. They may affect just one side of the face (unilateral) or both (bilateral). The problems are sometimes present with other congenital problems, for example heart defects or malformations of the brain. The failure of the palate (the roof of the mouth) to fuse during development can lead to problems with feeding during early life as milk escapes into the nasal passages. The muscles that control swallowing (and later on, speech) can be affected. The clefts can usually be repaired surgically, although problems with speech production might continue.

Children with cleft lip and palate usually have the corrective surgery completed preschool (see the advice in *Disfigurement and difference*). Residual problems can result in difficulty with speech, in which case working with a speech and language therapist is very important. School-based *Interdisciplinary working* might be necessary for some children, while community medical services will manage others. Effective links with parents and good pastoral arrangements will provide support for these children. The advice in *Speech and language problems* will apply. It is unlikely that the curriculum should be modified for children because they have a cleft lip and palate.

Useful links
CLAPA
235–237 Finchley Road
London NW3 6LS
Tel: 020 7431 0033
Fax 020 7431 8881
E-mail: info@clapa.com
www.clapa.com

Clumsy child syndrome *see* Dyspraxia

Coarctation of the aorta

Coarctation of the aorta is the name given to a congenital narrowing of the main blood vessel after it leaves the heart. The condition can vary in severity from being so slight as to be undetectable through to critical narrowing that threatens the baby's life or causes complete interruption to the aorta. This narrowing means that the heart has to work much harder than normal to pump blood around the body. Severe coarctation causes symptoms in newborn babies and in infants. Less severe cases may go unnoticed in childhood, although they lead to high blood pressure. An operation is usually required to treat the condition. This condition can coexist with other heart defects (see *Congenital heart diseases*).

Cochlear implant

Cochlear implant is a specialised implanted device that converts sound into electrical impulses, which can then be interpreted by the brain as sound. It is used for certain children with severe hearing loss. The systems vary slightly but generally include a microphone, a speech processor, a transmitter link and a fully implantable device containing an electronics package.

Children with cochlear implants can be educated in mainstream and special schools. They will be subject to close medical monitoring and regular hearing tests by professionals from supporting services. School-based *Interdisciplinary working* involving specialist teachers, audiologists and audio technicians will be necessary. Effective links with parents and good pastoral arrangements will provide support for these children. Staff in school will need to support children in the management of their equipment. In order to ensure the best performance from the implant, it is important to develop excellent and dependable means of communicating with parents. A good strategy for home and school is to rapidly develop rapidly the child's independence in management of the implant. The younger child will need more assistance and support but by secondary school it would be reasonable to expect independence other than in extreme circumstances. It is sensible to have spare batteries and leads available in school; batteries last longer if stored in a cool place or the fridge.

The microphone is extremely important; a directional microphone will filter out the other sounds and this allows the child to hear the teacher much better. It may be possible to have more than one microphone available for staff. Technical advice might be needed to get the best possible arrangement in classrooms and other areas in school. As static electricity can impair the performance of the implant and possibly cause damage, it is important to be aware of those parts of the school that seem to produce static – most children will know where these are. Finding areas of the school that produce static can be a good science-related topic. It will also help if parents choose clothing that does not produce static. If the child has to go on slides or large playground equipment where friction is possible, make sure he or she removes the processor. Very small children need to be made to wear their processor in a place where it is least likely to get damaged and parents will usually have sorted out a weatherproof bag that can be 'locked'. It is important that the processor does not get wet or sandy. The implant can be broken in a heavy fall; however, this is unlikely as they are quite robust.

Children's access to the curriculum should be monitored and modified accordingly; the advice of specialist teachers for the hearing impaired will be helpful. For the child who is reading, ensure that close captioning/subtitles are on TV and videos, as this assists in the learning of speech and the learning of the sounds of letters and vowels. It is gener-

ally better to place the child with a cochlear implant in the middle of the classroom rather than right at the front, because it is important for the child to be able to hear the responses of other children to the rear as well as to the front and not to be dominated by the volume of the teacher's speech. It is a good idea to help other children get to know about the implant and to learn the best tones and speeds of speaking.

Useful links
Royal National Institute for Deaf People
19–23 Featherstone Street
London EC1Y 8SL
Tel: 020 7296 8000
E-mail: informationline@rnid.org.uk
www.rnid.org.uk/index.htm

Coeliac disease

Coeliac disease is caused by intolerance to gluten in the diet. Gluten is in many foods, for instance bread, biscuits and other foods containing wheat. The symptoms are of diarrhoea, weight loss (or failure to gain weight normally), abdominal pain and bloating. Children are often also miserable. The condition sometimes runs in families. The disease is treated by avoiding gluten in the diet. A very small number of children with coeliac disease can have an itchy skin rash known as dermatitis herpetiformis – this can affect elbows, buttocks and knees.

Children with coeliac disease can be educated in mainstream and special schools. The extent to which coeliac disease affects schooling depends on how children have learned to manage their dietary needs. Some children with coeliac disease can have difficulties sticking to their strict diet at school and lapses are not uncommon. School-based *Interdisciplinary working* might be necessary for some children, while community medical services will manage others. Effective links with parents and good pastoral arrangements will provide support for these children. Those children with dermatitis herpetiformis may need support with some dressings. Children in the primary phase may need special attention – they might not tell staff when there is discomfort or a problem with a dressing for their dermatitis because they are engrossed in a particular activity or because they may prefer to avoid treatment. Special arrangements will probably be needed to provide access to some sporting activities – swimming is possible but medical advice will probably be necessary.

Children with coeliac disease have a condition that if well managed is unlikely to effect their education.

Useful links
British Association of Dermatologists
19 Fitzroy Square
London W1T 6EH
Tel: 020 7383 0266
Fax: 020 7388 5263
E-mail: admin@bad.org.uk
www.skinhealth.co.uk/contact/index.htm

Coeliac Society
PO Box 220
High Wycombe HP11 2HY
Tel: 01494 437278
Fax 01494 474349
E-mail: publications@coeliac.co.uk
www.coeliac.co.uk

Coloboma

Coloboma is a notch, fold or fissure that occurs as the eye forms during early development of the fetus. It may be noticed as a notch in the eyelid or an abnormally shaped pupil. It might cause no difficulties in some while in others it can cause complete visual loss, particularly if the retina is involved as part of the malformation.

Children with coloboma can be educated in mainstream and special schools. School-based *Interdisciplinary working* might be necessary for some children, while community medical services will manage others. For further advice see *Visual impairment* and *Blindness*. The child's appearance can be adversely affected (see *Disfigurement and difference.*)

Children with coloboma can sometimes have other problems such as learning difficulties or behaviour problems. Occasionally there are more severe problems or disorders. Children with coloboma often have a dislike to strong light (photophobia) because the pupil can't react to light in the normal way. Tinted glasses may be recommended. Some children with coloboma may need a highly specialised curriculum.

Useful links
Hands and Eyes
A USA specialist teacher maintains this useful online newsletter for teachers and caregivers of visually impaired students and their friends. It includes art, cooking and manipulative activities that visually impaired students can do individually or in small groups. It is for teachers and support staff in need of ideas for classroom activities and is particularly useful for pupils with multiple impairments such as developmental disability and motor impairment.
www.home.earthlink.net/~vharris/

RNIB Education Information Services
224 Great Portland Street
London W1N 6AA
Tel: 020 7388 1266
E-mail: webmaster@rnib.org.uk
www.rnib.org.uk
RNIB's curriculum information service offers information and advice to all professionals supporting a visually impaired child in mainstream or special schools.
www.rnib.org.uk/curriculum/
RNIB's accessing technology pages provide information about applications of technology in employment, at study and in leisure.
www.rnib.org.uk/technology/

V.I. Guide
This site contains information on many topics relating to parenting and teaching a child with visual impairments.
www.viguide.com/

Conduct disorder or disruptive behaviour disorder

Conduct disorder or disruptive behaviour disorder is when children exhibit persistently antisocial behaviour. It often takes the form of physically destructive behaviour and does not respond to the usual measures that normally control aberrant behaviour. Children with this problem often also have learning difficulties and low self-esteem. It is generally preceded by the less severe and descriptive condition known as oppositional defiant disorder. It is important for staff in school to be aware when hostility and defiance become the rule rather than the exception. The extreme antisocial symptoms of conduct disorder cannot be ignored by a

school and can be particularly disruptive. School-based *Interdisciplinary working* including skilled child mental health workers, child mental health teams and therapists can be helpful. Once the condition is confirmed a whole-school approach to working with the child will be needed and set out in a detailed plan that includes high levels of collaboration between home and school.

With early intervention, a skilled team and sufficient time to understand the child, much help can be given. Where conduct disorder becomes ingrained and long-standing it can be very difficult to manage. It can be difficult to find out what is going on with some children – diagnosis at times can move through a number of possibilities including mood disorders, psychotic disorders, *ADHD* and impairments associated with other conditions. It is not unusual for there to be uncertainty in establishing precise diagnoses; this should not deter the school in providing the very best in counselling, pastoral support and behavioural management.

Useful links
Association for Workers with Children with Emotional and Behavioural Difficulties
Administrative Officer
Charlton Court
East Sutton
Maidstone ME17 3DQ
Tel: 01622 843104
E-mail: awcebd@mistral.co.uk
www.awcebd.co.uk./contact/index.htm

Behaviour Change Consultancy
24 Rochdale
Harold Road
London SE19 3TF

Tel: 020 8653 9768

E-mail: bcc@behaviourchange.com

www.behaviourchange.com/index.htm

TEAM TEACH

Tel: 01403 268928

E-mail: George@team-teach.co.uk

www.team-teach.co.uk/index.html

Training in positive handling strategies through a holistic approach to managing difficult, disturbing, and sometimes dangerous behaviours. This provides the least intrusive positive handling strategy and a continuum of gradual and graded techniques.

Conductive education

Conductive education is a holistic approach to the education of children who have neurological impairment resulting in weak or uncoordinated movement (see *Cerebral palsy*). Conductive education was developed in Budapest by Dr Andras Peto (1900–1967), a physician, educator and visionary. Peto's work is based on the adaptability of the human brain and its ability to create new or other paths to the spinal cord. Conductive education helps find the best route from brain to limb allowing successful motor control.

Sessions are led by a conductor trained in all aspects of physical, intellectual, social, emotional and psychological development. Each child is seen as a whole human being and progress is continually monitored. The conductor sets individual goals that are broken down into smaller tasks that are key to basic functional movements such as rolling, stretching and bending limbs, closing and opening hands, and sitting with a straight back. Using commands and songs, the conductor prepares each child; the task is then carried out to rhythmical counting, singing or music. In this way, the conductor orchestrates all of the child's learning by integrating movement with communication, cognition and sensory learning while at the same time developing independence. The conductor is responsible for motivating the children to become active participants in their learning and to complete their tasks successfully. The intensity of exercises builds both physical stamina and independence.

Sessions take place in small groups where children can see and be motivated by the success of each other. They work with simple wood furniture that is ideal for grasping, pushing and pulling. For example, a ladder-back chair is used for pulling-up to stand, and then for pushing to walk.

Children learn the capacity to solve the problems of daily living from dressing, eating and self-help, through to living independently. Children with motor disabilities are taught to see themselves very positively as young people who can succeed. The specific movements and structure of the daily physical routine are designed to promote muscle and bone development. For example, weight bearing while walking encourages the correct formation of hip joints, legs and feet.

In the UK there are a number of 'Schools for Parents' taking children from 6 months to 5 years who have been diagnosed with a neurological impairment such as cerebral palsy. In a small number of education authorities, special schools provide conductive education. By participating in classes with their children, parents learn management techniques that enable them to support their children's development. Parents in turn draw strength from the positive, lively and structured sessions, and they see their children enjoying learning and making progress. Routines and sequences can be built into life at home thus providing children with integrated support.

Useful links
National Institute of Conductive Education
Cannon Hill House
Russell Road
Birmingham B13 8RD
Tel: 0121 449 1569
E-mail: foundation@conductive-educa-tion.org.uk
www.conductive-education.org.uk

Conductive hearing loss

Conductive hearing loss is deafness caused by any problem that affects the sounds entering the ear, vibrating the eardrum or transmitting the vibrations to the auditory nerve. This can be due to wax or foreign bodies lodged in the ear canal, middle ear infection (see *Otitis media*) or diseases that affect the bones of the middle ear. Many children will experience some kind of conductive hearing loss at some time during their education. Some inherited conditions are very likely to bring conductive hearing loss, e.g. *Down's syndrome, Noonan syndrome, Treacher Collins syndrome.*

Whatever the reason that prevents sound from reaching the functioning inner ear, the impact on a child's learning of language and education can be significant. Children with conductive hearing loss can be educated in mainstream and special schools. School-based *Interdisciplinary working* involving specialist teachers, audiologists and audio technicians might be necessary for some children, while community medical services will manage others. Effective links with parents and good pastoral arrangements will provide support for these children. The advice found under *Hearing impairment* will apply.

Conditions of a short duration should be monitored and will need basic attention, such as not placing children where there is noisy equipment or making sure that they are sitting near the teacher. It is also helpful to check systematically for understanding and learning, making sure children see those who are speaking and ensuring those who speak do so clearly. Should a child's speech become lazy and unclear, staff should contact parents recommending a visit to their general practitioner for possible referral to the audiologist to check hearing, or to the speech and language therapist. Longer-term conditions may require *Hearing aids*. It is useful to recognise that children with fluctuating conductive hearing loss can present with classroom behaviour problems and might appear not to be paying attention.

Congenital heart diseases

These are a group of conditions where the child is born with heart problems that developed as the heart itself formed (see under specific entries: *Atrial septal defect; Atrioventricular septal defect; Coarctation of the aorta; Hypoplastic left heart; Patent ductus arteriosus; Pulmonary stenosis; Pulmonary atresia;*

Tachyarrhythmia; *Tachycardia*; *Tetralogy of Fallot*; *Tricuspid atresia*; and *Ventricular septal defect*.

Congenital heart conditions have consequences for children's education and lifestyle. Because there is a very wide range of congenital heart conditions, the degree and complexity means that no child can be treated in the same way as another. Some children with congenital heart conditions may not be able to have corrective surgery. The extent to which heart disease affects schooling depends on how children manage the symptoms of their condition and the medical treatments and/or interventions required. Some children will need heart or heart and lung transplantation and this need for transplantation presents many difficulties, with painful decisions for both the recipient and donor parents. When any surgery is needed, children can be educated by the hospital school or service; it is very important to have effective channels of communication between the child's local school and hospital school in order to provide continuity of curriculum.

Children with heart conditions can be educated in mainstream and special schools. School-based *Interdisciplinary working* might be necessary for some children, while others will have their condition managed by hospital and community medical services. Effective links with parents and good pastoral arrangements will provide support for these children.

Children with heart disease will need access to the same curriculum as their peers. Children who have not had their condition corrected can tire more quickly than other children. They should be allowed

to stop when they feel like it. Classmates should be appropriately informed of their classmate's condition and its consequences. Many of these children will become breathless more quickly and their lips and skin can become blue. In some conditions the child looks normal but still cannot keep up with his or her peers, and will need rest from time to time. Staff should be aware of the things that they can do in the event of children showing distress or discomfort. At break times children should be given the opportunity to stay in a warm place. A school needs good systems of support and opportunities for children to catch up after periods of absence. Children needing frequent absence from school and time-consuming treatments can lead to staff having low expectations of them and school friendships will be disrupted. It is important to explore all possible ways of supporting children who are absent for long periods and to provide a range of ways to help them catch up with work; this becomes very important where children are mid-syllabus for externally accredited examinations.

Children in the primary phase may need special attention, as they might not anticipate a problem or they might become engrossed in a particular activity and not know how to moderate it. It can be very difficult to persuade a young active child not to do the same as their classmates. Pupils in the secondary phase will want to be as independent as their contemporaries – they may need support in explaining to others how they need to behave differently. In most cases children with heart conditions will limit their own activity without restriction from an adult; if this is not the case seek advice from the medical team. Children might not be able to take part in contact sports, and special arrangements will then be needed to give access to appropriate sports. Alternative sporting activities such as archery, ballroom dancing, ballet, bowls, 10-pin bowling, cricket, croquet, fishing, golf, gentle cycling, orienteering, sailing or pony trekking could be offered instead. The safety measures for all pupils are generally sufficient. Overall children with heart disease have a condition that might at times significantly interfere with their education.

Useful links
The Association for Children with Heart Disorders (England & Wales)
26 Elizabeth Drive
Helmshore
Rossendale BB4 4JB
Tel: 01706 213632
E-mail: information@tachd.org.uk

The Association for Children with Heart Disorders (Scotland)
Killieard House
Killiecrankie
Pitlochry PH16 5LN
Tel: 01796 473204
E-mail: information@tachd.org.uk
www.tachd.org.uk

British Heart Foundation
14 Fitzhardinge Street
London W1H 6DH
Tel: 020 7935 0185
E-mail: Internet@bhf.org.uk
www.bhf.org.uk

Children's Heart Federation
52–54 Kennington Oval
London SE11 5SW
Tel: 0808 808 5000
E-mail: chf@dircon.co.uk
www.childrens-heart-fed.org.uk

ECHO (Evelina Children's Heart Organisation)
Wild Flowers
Pett Road
Pett Village
Hastings TN35 4EY
Tel: 01424 813785

Grown Up Congenital Heart (GUCH) Patients Association
12 Rectory Road
Stanford-le-Hope SS17 0DL
E-mail: info@guch.org
www.guch.demon.co.uk

HeartLine Association
Community Link
Surrey Heath House
Knoll Road
Camberley GU15 3HH
Tel: 01276 707636
E-mail: heartline@easynet.co.uk
www.heartline.org.uk

Heart Link
68 Rockhill Drive
Mountsorrel
Leicester LE12 7DT
Tel: 0500 382152
www.heartlink-glenfield.org.uk

Heart Transplant Families Together
c/o Cardiomyopathy Association

40 The Metro Centre
Watford WD1 8SB
Tel: 01923 249977

Left Heart Matters
c/o 24 Calthorpe Road
Edgbaston
Birmingham B15 1RP
Tel: 0121 455 8982
E-mail: info@lhm.org.uk

Young at Heart
5 Orchard Close
Handsworth
Birmingham B21 9PH
Tel: 0121 523 7840
E-mail: support@youngatheart.org.uk
www.youngatheart.org.uk

Conjunctivitis

Conjunctivitis is inflammation of the thin transparent membrane that covers the surface of the eyeball and the lining of the eyelid. It causes redness, soreness and a feeling of grittiness. Pus will also often discharge from the corner of the eye or can cause the eyelids to stick together. The condition can be caused by bacteria, viruses or allergies (for instance to pollens – this is called vernal conjunctivitis). Chemicals, dust and bigger foreign bodies can also cause similar problems. When infection is suspected as a cause of the conjunctivitis, contact with others at school should be avoided until the infection has cleared up. Treatment of infections is usually with antibiotic drops or ointments placed directly onto the eye. Children with this condition can experience pain, discomfort and temporarily impaired vision. Because in some instances it is extremely contagious, good hygiene is vital to prevent spread and it is very important to check that all children wash their hands well. It is unlikely that the curriculum should be modified for children because they have conjunctivitis.

Constipation

Constipation is the term given to the passage of hard infrequent stools. It is quite common in children. In most children there is no underlying serious problem with the bowel itself and treatment is with increasing the amount of fluid and fibre in the diet. Laxatives are often prescribed. Children with severe constipation may get what is known as overflow diarrhoea. Here the child unwittingly passes liquid faeces, often into their underwear. Other pupils may tease and the child can quickly lose confidence and self-esteem. Low self-esteem might in turn worsen the existing continence difficulties. Treatment is often required for a considerable period of time (years). Some children pass faeces into their underwear without suffering from constipation, or hide the stool in an inappropriate place; this is known as encopresis.

Cortical blindness

Cortical blindness occurs when the eye functions as an organ for focusing and transmitting images but the brain appears unable to interpret the information. This can follow head injury, insult to the developing brain (see *Cerebral palsy*) or infection. The visual function will often improve a little with time, but for most children it means greatly reduced vision. There can be other difficulties as the condition often occurs together with other medical and developmental problems. Similar problems can be encountered in children suffering from delayed visual maturation, although vision can improve as the child develops.

Children with cortical blindness can be educated in mainstream and special schools. School-based *Interdisciplinary working* will be necessary including the advice of a specialist teacher for visual impairment in the planning of an effective educational programme.

Vision loss can be from mild to severe, temporary or permanent. The visual acuity of children with cortical blindness can fluctuate within a short period of time for no obvious reason, and because of this staff need to be vigilant and have rapid access to a specialist teacher for visual impairment. A child might be able to see an object one day and be unable to see it the next. Spatial confusion is common; for example being unable to find things even though they can see them. They may also be visually inattentive and not want to look at objects, preferring their sense of touch. It is not unusual to see a child turn their head away as they explore an object with their hands. A child may have better peripheral than central vision and thus look at objects out of the side of their eye. They may have visual field losses that are not symmetrical (one eye might be worse than the other). Children with cortical blindness experience problems with specific types of visual tasks such as figure-ground differentiation

(seeing an object instead of the background), and with complex visual displays with many elements. It is better to select materials, pictures and displays with one or two subjects on a strongly contrasted background. For some children access to a darkened sensory room is invaluable. In this setting, presentations can be specially lit and children can practise and develop tracking and scanning skills. For further advice see *Visual impairment*.

Useful links
Hands and Eyes
A USA specialist teacher maintains this useful online newsletter for teachers and caregivers of visually impaired students and their friends. It includes art, cooking and manipulative activities that visually impaired students can do individually or in small groups. It is for teachers and support staff in need of ideas for classroom activities and is particularly useful for pupils with multiple impairments such as developmental disability and motor impairment.
www.home.earthlink.net/~vharris/
RNIB Education Information Services
224 Great Portland Street
London W1N 6AA
Tel: 020 7388 1266
E-mail: webmaster@rnib.org.uk
www.rnib.org.uk
RNIB's curriculum information service offers information and advice to all professionals supporting a visually impaired child in mainstream or special schools.
www.rnib.org.uk/curriculum/
RNIB's accessing technology pages provide information about applications of technology in employment, at study and in leisure.
www.rnib.org.uk/technology/

V.I. Guide
This site contains information on many topics relating to parenting and teaching a child with visual impairments.
www.viguide.com/

Cough

Cough is heard when there is sudden breathing out against closed vocal cords, which then open, explosively releasing air. It is an effective way of removing unwanted debris from the breathing tubes that transmit air into the lungs. Coughs occur with (and following) infections and with allergies.

Children with coughs can be educated in mainstream and special schools. The extent to which coughs etc. affect schooling depends on the severity of the symptom or underlying condition and the medical interventions required. These conditions are usually simply managed by community medical services. Effective links with parents and good pastoral arrangements might be needed.

Children with coughs should not need different curriculum arrangements to their peers. Staff should be aware of the supportive things that they can do where there are allergies. Some families will want to explore diets excluding certain foods, and schools can help parents by managing access to permitted foods and supervising snacks at break times and by observing children over time.

Useful links
Action against Allergy
PO Box 278
Twickenham TW1 4QQ
Tel: 020 8892 2711

E-mail:
AAA@actionagainstallergy.freeserve.co.uk
www.actionagainstallergy.co.uk

Breathe Easy
British Lung Foundation
78 Hatton Garden
London EC1N 8LD
Tel: 020 7831 5831
E-mail: blf@britishlungfoundation.com
www.lunguk.org

British Allergy Foundation
Deepdene House
30 Bellegrove Road
Welling DA16 3PY
Tel: 020 8303 8583
E-mail: info@allergyfoundation.com
www.allergyfoundation.com

National Society for Research into Allergies and Environmental Diseases
PO Box 45
Hinckley LE10 1JY
Tel/Fax: 01455 250715
E-mail: nsra.allergy@virgin.net

Cranial nerve palsies

Cranial nerve palsies are weaknesses of muscles or groups of muscles in the head and neck that are supplied by nerves emanating from the brain (most nerves emerge from the spinal cord). Cranial nerve palsies affecting the production of speech, result in abnormal speech sounds, or can restrict the ability to speak altogether (see *Alternative and augmentative communication*). Some children are born with cranial nerve palsies, while in others it occurs after injury, infection or from other causes within the brain.

Children with cranial nerve palsies have their educational needs met in mainstream and special schools. The extent to which cranial nerve palsies will affect schooling can vary significantly. School-based *Interdisciplinary working* including the speech and language therapist might be necessary for some children, others will have their condition managed by community medical services. Effective links with parents and good pastoral arrangements will provide support for these children. For further advice see *Speech and language problems*.

Overall children with cranial nerve palsies have a condition that will to some extent affect their communication and subsequently their education.

Cri du chat syndrome

Cri du chat syndrome is caused by a loss of genetic material from the 5th chromosome. It causes growth problems, a small head (*Microcephaly*), low muscle tone and a weak, cat-like cry (in early life). There are also developmental problems and later on learning difficulties. Head banging and other self-injury can occur in later childhood.

Most children with cri du chat syndrome require a highly differentiated curriculum. Generally children are delayed in all areas of learning and require an educational programme designed and monitored by a multidisciplinary team (see *Interdisciplinary working* in Chapter 3). Children do make progress but at a slower rate than their peers. Significant attention should be given to communication as many children have little

or no speech. A communication programme should be devised with advice from a speech and language therapist – this might include the use of gestures, signing, symbols and picture communication systems. Some children will benefit from *Alternative and augmentative communication* devices. Support and assistance will be needed in the classroom to provide the child with access to the curriculum. As many children have a short attention span, a number of relevant activities need to be prepared to keep the child interested. Some children can exhibit self-injurious behaviour and will require a behaviour management plan.

Useful links
Cri du Chat Syndrome Support Group
7 Penny Lane
Barwell
Leicester LE9 8HJ
Tel: 01455 841680
E-mail: cdcssg@yahoo.co.uk
www.cridchat.u-net.com

Crohn's disease

Crohn's disease is a chronic inflammatory disease that can affect any portion of the gut from the mouth down to the anus. The symptoms can be of loose, bloody, mucous-filled stools and abdominal pain or discomfort. Children might not grow adequately and the diarrhoea and pain can interfere with normal school activities. They can also become lethargic and tire easily. It is a disease punctuated by periods of remission from the disease and then exacerbations. Some children have arthritis, eye problems and rashes associated with the condition. Treatment is with drugs by mouth; in some children a special diet (elemental) is recommended. Sometimes surgery is required.

Children with Crohn's disease can be educated in mainstream and special schools. School-based *Interdisciplinary working* might be necessary for some children, while community medical services will manage others. Effective links with parents and good pastoral arrangements will provide support for these children.

Some children with Crohn's disease need special arrangements to get to toilets when they need to and need to rest in a room that is quiet at break and lunch times. It is unlikely that the curriculum should be modified for children because of the disease.

Useful links
Crohn's in Childhood Research Association
Parkgate House
356 West Barnes Lane
Motspur Park KT3 6NB
Tel: 020 8949 6209
E-mail: support@cicra.org
www.cicra.org

National Association for Colitis and Crohn's Disease
PO Box 205
St Albans AL1 1AB
**www.digestivedisorders.org.uk/leaflets/coli
tis.html**

Croup

Croup is a viral infection affecting the larynx,

vocal cords and windpipe (trachea). It occurs in younger children and causes a characteristic barking cough and noisy breathing. The infection is usually mild and gets better without specific treatment, although more serious cases can be treated with steroids. More severely affected children will require admission to hospital and very severely affected children might need help with their breathing (ventilation on an intensive care unit).

This condition is usually managed by family doctors and could include time in hospital or the interventions of community medical services. Effective links with parents and good pastoral arrangements might be needed. It is unlikely that the curriculum should be modified for children because they have croup; however, a very small number of children will be absent from school while receiving treatment.

Crouzon's syndrome

Crouzon's syndrome is a rare syndrome affecting the development of the skull and face. This leads to the child having unusual-looking facial features and shallow eye sockets, which make the eyes look protuberant. The skull problems can lead to increased pressure on the developing brain, which can, in turn, lead to learning difficulties and can threaten vision. Treatment is with a multidisciplinary medical and surgical team working from a specialised craniofacial surgery unit.

Children with Crouzon's syndrome require the close attention of a highly skilled medical team throughout their school years. Careful *Interdisciplinary working* is necessary to provide support advice and counselling. Prolonged admissions to hospital are likely and close liaison with hospital schools and/or outreach services can help provide continuity of the curriculum. A school needs good systems of support and opportunities for children to catch up after periods of absence. This becomes very important where children are mid-syllabus for externally accredited examinations. Children needing frequent absence from school and time-consuming treatments can lead to staff having low expectations of them and school friendships will be disrupted.

Periodic surgical treatment to ears and eyes can cause fluctuations in sensory acuity. Some children will experience problems related to their increasing physical differences, and care and encouragement is needed in all settings. Children will be very different in appearance; this should be dealt with sensitively by all staff, particularly in informal settings such as the playground (see *Disfigurement and difference*).

Useful links
Headlines – the Craniofacial Support Group
44 Helmsdale Road
Leamington Spa CV32 7DW
Tel: 01926 334629
E-mail: SteveMoody@headlines.org.uk
www.headlines.org.uk

Cushing's syndrome

Cushing's syndrome is most often seen in children who are prescribed long-term steroids because of illnesses such as renal disease, chronic lung disease of prematurity or asthma. It causes growth failure and weight gain, making the child short but rela-tively obese. There can be bruising, *Osteoporosis*, high blood pressure and behavioural changes. Sometimes it is due to a tumour of the adrenal gland (a gland located just above the kidneys), which secretes the body's own steroids. It can also be due to disease of the pituitary gland (located at the base of the brain).

When the adrenal gland does not produce adequate amounts of steroid, the child may have hypoadrenalism. This causes problems with low blood pressure, low blood sugar and the salt balance in the blood. Sometimes it occurs as part of a condition known as congenital adrenal hyperplasia (which can also affect the gender of the child – see *Ambiguous genitalia*). Treatment is with oral (by mouth) replacement steroids.

Children with Cushing's syndrome can be educated in mainstream and special schools. School-based *Interdisciplinary working* might be necessary for some children, while community medical services will manage others. Effective links with parents and good pastoral arrangements will provide support for these children. Some children can look different and therefore might need additional care (see *Disfigurement and difference*). Where there is muscular wastage of the limbs, *Osteoporosis* (fragility of the bones) and/or high blood pressure, the advice of medical professionals might be needed to ensure that exercises, activities and games in PE are appropriate.

Useful links
Val Howarth
Cushing Care
Meadows, Woodplumpton Village
Preston PR4 0LJ
Tel/Fax: 01772 690680

Cystic fibrosis

Cystic fibrosis is an inherited condition that makes the secretions of the lung and pancreas excessively viscous. The result is long-term lung infections that damage the developing lung and cause difficulties in absorbing food from the gut. The lung infections are treated with antibiotics, chest physiotherapy and inhaled medications. The poor absorption of food is treated by taking pancreatic enzyme supplements with meals and snacks. The progressive lung damage means that the condition is life limiting, although lung transplantation and heart–lung transplantation have recently become available for some individuals. Older children and teenagers with the condition can also develop diabetes and liver disease.

Children with cystic fibrosis can be educated in mainstream and special schools. The extent to which cystic fibrosis affects schooling will vary for each child. Community medical services or specialist cystic fibrosis teams including a physiotherapist usually help manage this condition (see *Interdisciplinary working* in chapter 3). Effective links with parents and good pastoral arrangements will be needed.

Children with cystic fibrosis will need access to the same curriculum as their peers, although frequent absence from school is likely due to chest infections. A school needs good systems of support and opportunities for children to catch up after periods of absence; this becomes very important where children are mid-syllabus for externally accredited examinations. Children needing frequent absence from school and time-consuming treatments can lead to staff having low expectations of them and school friendships will be disrupted.

Staff will need to have high expectations and be aware of the things that are needed to support children and keep them healthy. Some children will have severe coughing attacks, occasionally coughing up mucus and sometimes vomiting. The physical management of this is important but also the way that the remainder of the class accept this difference will matter. Physiotherapy sessions should be built into the school day with the minimum disruption to the curriculum; it may be possible for these to take place at break times. Younger children might need help with chest physiotherapy while older children are often able to do their own. A separate room or area will be needed for physiotherapy. Medications should be given according to locally agreed policy. Special consideration is needed for sporting activities as, although physical exercise is beneficial, some children can seem lethargic following illness. Overall children with cystic fibrosis have a condition that will interfere with their education and need special consideration.

Useful links
Breathe Easy
British Lung Foundation
78 Hatton Garden, London EC1N 8LD
Tel: 020 7831 5831
E-mail: blf@britishlungfoundation.com
www.lunguk.org

Cystic Fibrosis Trust
11 London Road, Bromley BR1 1BY
Tel: 020 8464 7211
E-mail: enquiries@cftrust.org.uk
www.cftrust.org.uk

Cystitis *see* Urinary tract infection

D

Daytime wetting

Daytime (diurnal) wetting occurs because of immaturity, problems with the nerves that control the bladder and its sphincter (see *Neuropathic bladder*), bladder irritability, urine infections and occasionally behavioural difficulties; therefore treatment can be behavioural, developmental or medical. For the child with diurnal wetting, these problems can lead to blame at home, bullying at school (if the child smells of stale urine) and thereby to low self-esteem.

Children who wet themselves have their educational needs met in mainstream and special schools. School-based *Interdisciplinary working* might be necessary for some children, while community medical services will manage others. Effective links with parents and good pastoral arrangements will provide support for these children.

Where staff are aware that children are wetting during the school day and that these are not 'accidents', then special care arrangements might be needed in order to manage the situation effectively without attracting unnecessary attention of peers. As wetting is very obvious, staff will need to develop ways of monitoring children to prevent inappropriate comments and/or bullying. It is unlikely that the curriculum should be modified for children because they are wetting during the school day, but measures may be needed to prevent adverse reactions that lead to low self-esteem and poor school work.

Useful links
Bedwetting.co.uk
4 Harforde Court
John Tate Road
Hertford SG13 7NW
Tel: 01992 526300
E-mail: info@bedwetting.co.uk
www.bedwetting.co.uk/nhsnews.htm

The Enuresis Resource & Information Centre
34 Old School House
Britannia Road
Kingswood
Bristol BS15 8DB
Tel: 0117 960 3060
E-mail: info@eric.org.uk
www.enuresis.org.uk

Deafblind

Deafblind is an impairment of both hearing and sight. Premature birth and birth trauma are now more common causes of congenital deafblindness. These can be associated with rare genetic disorders such as *CHARGE association* and *Usher syndrome* or with infections during pregnancy such as rubella. In addition, severe infections during early childhood such as *Meningitis* can lead to severe damage to the brain causing loss of sight and hearing. Children learn about themselves and nearly everything else through sight and hearing. Without these two senses, mobility, communication and learning are greatly affected. Deafblind children do not have sufficient sight or hearing to compensate for the other sense. They are unable to learn and function in the same way deaf or blind children can. Many children have other disabilities such as *Epilepsy*, feeding problems and severe physical disabilities.

Children who are deafblind can be educated in mainstream and special schools. In 1989 the Department of Education and Science (DES) published a Policy Statement *Educational Provision for Deafblind Children*, which acknowledged the use of the term 'deafblind' in the educational context and described the continuum of sensory loss as:

> a heterogeneous group of children who can suffer from varying degrees of visual and hearing impairment, perhaps combined with learning difficulties and physical disabilities, which can cause severe communication, developmental and educational problems. A precise description is difficult because the degrees of deafness and blindness, possibly combined with different degrees of other disabilities, are not uniform, and the educational needs of each child will have to be decided individually.

School-based *Interdisciplinary working* including specialist teachers and a specialist educational psychologist will be necessary. Effective links with parents and good pastoral arrangements will be needed to provide the child with support. Deafblind children need highly specialised support at the earliest possible age. Extreme isolation can lead to difficulties in communication and therefore the development of learning skills. The senses of touch and smell need to be developed to the full.

Developing communication skills is very important requiring intensive individual work. Children can be taught a range of communication systems including objects of reference, symbols, sign language and Braille. Many children will need an intervenor in order to access the world and to learn. A trained intervenor will motivate the child and become their eyes and ears providing feedback from the world. This complex role is necessary for deafblind children and requires high levels of skill and dedication.

In 1992 the Department for Education and Employment established a 3-year project to support the education of deafblind children. Follow-up work at the University of London Institute of Education funded by DfEE and Sense investigated the ways in which teachers enable deafblind pupils to access the school curriculum. The project looked at the impact of various types of training on teachers' perception of their lessons, pupil groupings and staff to pupil ratios, the content of the curriculum delivered, and the relationship between the National Curriculum and other curriculum approaches. (DfEE, Sense (1997) *Curriculum Access for Deafblind Children*.)

Useful links
Sense
11–13 Clifton Terrace
London N4 3SR
Tel: 020 7272 7774
E-mail: enquiries@sense.org.uk
www.sense.org.uk

Shared World Different Experiences: Designing the Curriculum for Pupils who are Deafblind (QCA/99/420) £6

www.deafblind.com/index.html#bsl

A Deafblindness Web Resource site owned and maintained by James Gallagher.

www.qca.org.uk/onq/schools/inclusion_wawn.asp

Deafness *see* Hearing impairment

Delayed visual maturation *see* Cortical blindness

Dermatitis herpstiformis *see* Coeliac diseases

Dermatomyositis

Dermatomyositis affects the skin and muscles causing inflammation. Joints can also be affected causing mobility problems. The muscles can be painful and weak. The muscles of the gut are sometimes affected and occasionally the child will have nodules of calcium under the skin. Treatment is with steroids and other immunosuppressing drugs during flare-ups of the condition.

Children with dermatomyositis can be educated in mainstream and special schools. The extent to which dermatomyositis affects schooling depends on the extent and activity of the condition and the medical interventions required. *Interdisciplinary working*, including the advice of a physiotherapist or occupational therapist, might be necessary for some children, while community medical services will manage others. Effective links with parents and good pastoral arrangements will provide support for these children.

Children will need access to the same curriculum as their peers although they can experience muscle weakness. All staff should be aware of the arrangements that should be in place so that children can receive treatment. Most children are knowledgeable about the way their disorder affects them and with support will deal with problems well.

Children in the primary phase will need special attention – they might not tell staff when they have a problem because they are engrossed in a particular activity or because they might prefer to avoid treatment. Particular measures may be needed where children are having physical problems. Fatigue and discomfort can mean that some children will require a quiet place to rest and shorter lessons. Overall children with dermatomyositis have a condition that can sometimes interfere with their education.

Useful links
British Association of Dermatologists
19 Fitzroy Square
London W1T 6EH
Tel: 020 7383 0266
Fax: 020 7388 5263
E-mail: admin@bad.org.uk
www.skinhealth.co.uk/contact/index.htm

Myositis Support Group
146 Newtown Road
Woolston
Southampton SO19 9HR
Tel: 023 8044 9708
E-mail: dpsg@dial.pipex.com
www.myositis.org.uk

Developmental coordination disorder *see* Dyspraxia

Developmental motor disability see Dyspraxia

Diabetes insipidus

Diabetes insipidus is a condition where the child is unable to concentrate the urine and is prone to rapid dehydration and salt imbalance. It can cause serious collapse if not treated. Some children with the condition fail to grow normally and some have concentration difficulties. Continence may be an issue in children whose treatment is inadequate (see *Neuropathic bladder*). In most cases medication is available to treat the condition.

Children with diabetes insipidus can be educated in mainstream and special schools. School-based *Interdisciplinary working* might be necessary for some children, although most will have their condition managed by community medical services and these arrangements will not adversely affect schooling. Effective links with parents and good pastoral arrangements will provide support for these children. Some children with diabetes insipidus might need special arrangements to get to toilets when they need to, and to fresh drinking water; they may also need to rest in a room that is quiet at break and lunch times. It is unlikely that the curriculum should be modified for children because they have diabetes insipidus; however, some children might need access to medication while at school.

Useful links
National Kidney Federation
6 Stanley Street
Worksop S81 7HX
Tel: 0845 601 0209

E-mail: helpline@kidney.org.uk
www.kidney.org.uk

Nephronline
E-mail: info@nephronline.org
www.nephronline.org/

Diabetes mellitus

Diabetes mellitus occurs when the child is unable to use sugar in the diet. Untreated children pass lots of urine and are very thirsty. They lose weight and can quickly become ill with vomiting, dehydration and may even become comatose. Treatment is generally with insulin injections and a diet that provides a predictable amount of sugar and carbohydrate. The injections are usually required several times per day, and may be required during the school day (for instance, before lunch). In treated diabetics, the blood sugar can fall too low causing hypoglycaemia (a 'hypo'). Hypos occur when insufficient food, or excessive exercise or insulin is taken. This might make the child sweaty, shaky, aggressive, slur their speech and might even result in a coma. Treatment is with sugar or other rapidly acting sources of carbohydrate. They may therefore need access to snacks or sugar as advised by their doctor during the school day. At times when children with diabetes have high blood sugar (hyperglycaemia), they must be allowed free access to water and to a quiet room where they can test their blood sugar or inject insulin, if necessary. Diabetic children can have emotional, eating, behavioural, and confidence difficulties as a result of their condition.

Children with diabetes can be educated in mainstream and special schools. Generally children will be learning how to manage their condition throughout their school years. School-based *Interdisciplinary working* might be necessary for some children, while community medical services will manage others. Effective links with parents and good pastoral arrangements will provide support for these children.

Where staff are aware that children are undergoing treatment for diabetes then consideration will need giving to ways in which they can be given the required support. It can be helpful to provide access to a quiet room where children can inject insulin. Children will need to check blood sugar levels at times during the day. Primary aged children may need adult supervision when checking blood sugar levels – this can happen away from the classroom but does not have to. Because exercise lowers blood sugar the advice of medical professionals might be needed to ensure that exercises, activities and games in PE are appropriate. Staff will need to keep a supply of emergency glucose on hand to treat hypoglycaemia. It is unlikely that the curriculum should be modified for children because they have diabetes. However it is possible that some measures will be needed to provide support and boost confidence.

Useful links
Diabetes UK Central Office
10 Queen Anne Street,
London W1G 9LH
Tel: 020 7323 1531
E-mail: info@diabetes.org.uk
www.diabetes.org.uk

Insulin Pumpers
www.insulin-pumpers.org.uk

DfES Publications Centre
PO Box 5050
Sudbury CO10 6ZQ
Tel: 0845 602 2260
www.dfes.gov.uk/medical/

Supporting Pupils with Medical Needs – a Good Practice Guide *is a document to help schools draw up policies on managing medication in schools, and to put in place effective management systems to support individual pupils with medical needs. This can be downloaded from DfES Website.*

JDRF Head Office
25 Gosfield Street
London W1W 6EB
Tel: 020 7436 3112
E-mail: info@jdrf.org.uk
www.jdrf.org.uk

Diarrhoea and vomiting

Diarrhoea and vomiting are usually signs of a gastrointestinal upset. Diarrhoea is excessively loose or watery stool, produced when the bowel empties more frequently than normal for the particular child. The upset can be caused by infections, inflammation, and malabsorption of food or stress. Gastrointestinal infections are usually viral and cause diarrhoea and vomiting for a few days. Bacterial infections also produce these symptoms and both bacterial and viral infections can occur as outbreaks within schools. Outbreaks might require investigation by public health doctors if food poisoning is suspected. In certain bowel conditions where the lining of the bowel is inflamed, diarrhoea and/or vomiting can result (see *Ulcerative colitis* and *Crohn's disease*). In conditions where the food is not absorbed properly by the bowel, the undigested food can pass rapidly through the bowel producing diarrhoea (see *Coeliac disease*). Stress and anxiety can cause the intestinal contents to hurry through the bowel producing diarrhoea. Occasionally vomiting can also occur. Where children have frequent episodes of diarrhoea, then links with parents and good pastoral arrangements will provide support for these children.

Most children will at some time experience diarrhoea or vomiting because of something that they have eaten. In most circumstances children stay at home and do not come to school until they are well. Where children are at school and become ill because of diarrhoea or vomiting, arrangements should be made for the child to be cared for while parents are contacted.

DiGeorge syndrome *see* Hypoparathyroidism

Diplegia *see* Cerebral palsy

Disfigurement and difference

Throughout the education system there are children and young people who are disfigured or different for some reason. Any disfigurement can lead to children experiencing social and psychological discomfort. It is very important for these children to be provided with appropriate support by the school's pastoral systems at all times. School-based staff may find it useful to develop good communication with parents and carers.

When children look different, they are greatly helped by being given school work that they can do well; the praise that follows promotes and sustains their self-esteem. They will benefit enormously from positive social and interpersonal skills – it is therefore helpful to support good friendship networks with children and staff whom affected children like and trust. Staff will need to find ways to help affected children to learn and cope with other people's reactions to them. It can be useful to explore perceptions of how a disfigured appearance or difference affects reactions and responses in others. Classes and perhaps the whole school can look at ways in which they could improve their understanding and thereby share positive experiences and learn ways of responding positively to the pupil who is disfigured or very different.

The responses of all people in the school to disfigurement or differences are important for obvious reasons. The messages given to a child with disfigurement or difference and to those who visit the school need to be positive. It is useful for staff to develop an understanding of what happens on a first meeting and what they could do to support both the pupil with a disfigurement and the new person. This kind of strategy depends on a range of interpersonal and social skills and a reasonable amount of confidence. It can be helpful to think of three steps in a process of social interaction that allow for information, give space for adjustment and move on to the next topic.

- *Stage One – Initial Reaction*: Extend and raise the awareness of staff so that they understand that when people first encounter someone who is significantly different in appearance, they nearly always react. This is natural, people cannot help themselves.
- *Stage Two – Respond Naturally*: Staff or the child need to respond naturally with enough information and reassurance to give the other person space to adjust. For example, a child may prefer to say 'I had an operation' to saying 'It's my cleft palate', or someone could say 'John had an operation because his palate was divided when he was born. He's fine again now.' It is a good idea to include the child because it is helpful to develop the capacity to respond naturally.
- *Stage Three – Move Attention Elsewhere*: It is a reasonably easy skill to learn how to move attention elsewhere to what was going on or away from the child's appearance. It is a good idea to have a number of things to say to move the situation on. For instance, 'Janet is recovering well, scars from operations are necessary. Have you ever had to have an operation?', or 'Ah yes, that's Philip's burn scar. He was burnt when he was seven. His pressure mask makes it hard for him to talk but he has no trouble hearing and understanding you. Come and look at the brilliant picture Philip did yesterday. Do you want to show your super picture Philip?' or, 'Adam's neurofibromatosis means that he does look different and is unable to use his left eye. He can see you with his right eye and understands what you are saying. Come and tell Adam what you think of his Geography Project work.' It is helpful to enable all staff, friends of the child and the child where possible to be able to move the attention of others from whatever it is about the child who looks different and on to something positive.

It is unlikely that the curriculum should be modified for children because they have a disfigurement or look very different.

Useful links
Changing Faces
1/2 Junction Mews
London W2 1PN
Tel: 020 7706 4232
E-mail: info@changingfaces.co.uk
www.cfaces.demon.co.uk

The Disfigurement Guidance Centre,
PO Box 7
Cupar KY15 4PF
Scotland
www.dgc.org.uk

Let's Face It Support Network
14 Fallowfield
Yateley
Camberley GU46 6LW
Tel: 01252 879630
E-mail: mike@letsfaceit.force9.net
www.letsfaceit.force9.co.uk

Down's syndrome

Down's syndrome is a congenital condition caused by having an extra copy of all, or part, of chromosome 21. Children usually have characteristic physical features. Many have other problems such as heart defects, bowel disorders (*Hirschsprung's bowel disease* and bowel blockages), *Visual impairments* (*Nystagmus, Cataracts*), *Hearing impairments* (*Conductive hearing loss* and deafness), orthopaedic problems such as atlanto-axial instability (instability of the neck vertebra), patella dislocation (displacement of the kneecap) and restricted growth. Subsequently they are at higher risk of *Leukaemia, Hypoadrenalism*, bacterial infections and, as adults, Alzheimer disease and coronary heart disease. It is one of the most early recognised causes of developmental delay and of learning difficulty, although the degree is variable.

The diagnosis of Down's syndrome is usually made soon after birth. Medical conditions such as bowel blockages or heart defects are usually treated early on in life. Delayed development is often apparent once any complicating medical conditions have been dealt with. Early input to maximise the child's development is helpful through preschool programmes such as 'Portage'. In the early years it is important to keep a close eye on vision, hearing, thyroid function and general neurological state.

Children may be anywhere on the learning spectrum and their educational needs will differ accordingly. Some might be cognitively delayed and need to spend longer than their peers in some subjects and areas of work. For many children there is a need for intensive work on speech, language and communication; school-based *Interdisciplinary working* will therefore include specialist teachers and/or speech and language therapists.

The exercise limitation associated with heart defects is generally 'self-regulated' by the child in that they will know when they are tired. However, it is important to check on indicators and the consequences of these with parents and medical advisers. In some cases all staff need to be aware of the warning signs and be able to implement appropriate strategies.

PE may need to be modified. Some older children can develop instability of the neck vertebrae (atlanto-axial instability), which has potentially serious neurological consequences. This limits some physical activities such as diving into water and forward rolls.

Useful links
Down's Syndrome Association
155 Mitcham Road
London SW17 9PG
Tel: 020 8682 4001
E-mail: info@downs-syndrome.org.uk
www.downs-syndrome.org.uk

The Scottish Down's Syndrome Association
158/160 Balgreen Road
Edinburgh EH11 3AU
Tel: 0131 313 4225
E-mail: info@sdsa.org.uk
www.dsscotland.org.uk

Dribbling

Dribbling is the overspill of saliva from the mouth. It is normal in infants and a proportion of young children will continue to dribble for the first few years. In many cases it appears to be related to the child's ability to control movements of the mouth and lips and hence is often more noticeable in children with speech and language delay.

Children who have difficulty with mouth control from motor problems such as *Cerebral palsy* may also dribble.

The condition improves in many children as development proceeds, although for older children this can be embarrassing and damage self-esteem. Drug treatments are of limited value, and surgery to reduce the amount of saliva produced could be offered to children with severe problems. The curriculum will not need to be modified for children because they dribble.

Dual sensory impairment *see* Deafblind

Duchenne muscular dystrophy

Duchenne muscular dystrophy (DMD) is a congenital condition affecting boys. It is caused by a defect in the gene that makes a protein that regulates muscle function. Boys with DMD can have delayed walking or present with excessive falling as toddlers; some have delayed speech. As the boys get older their muscles get weaker, despite looking abnormally big (pseudohypertrophy), and most are wheelchair-dependent by the time they reach the age of 10. Diagnosis is made by measuring muscle enzymes levels in the blood, specific genetic testing (blood tests), and looking at small specimens of muscle (muscle biopsy). Becker muscular dystrophy is a similar, although rarer, disease in which the same gene defect is present. The condition is, however, milder, and affected children may be able to walk until well into adult life.

Some boys have learning difficulties, but these are often mild. As the boys get older,

weakness gets more severe and dependency increases. Length of life is reduced, but quality of life can be maximised by providing environmental controls and medical or surgical treatments to minimise the effects of the increasing muscle weakness.

Boys with DMD can be educated in mainstream and special schools. School-based *Interdisciplinary working* involving a physiotherapist and an occupational therapist will eventually be necessary as boys get older. Effective links with parents and good pastoral arrangements will provide the family with support. The educational environment will need to link with the physical needs of the child and should include well-designed and spacious accommodation, as physical management of students becomes the priority.

Ideally boys should be taught in single-storey buildings with large classrooms and additional workspaces for therapist and medical teams. Specialised postural equipment might be needed together with equipment for lifting and transferring. High staffing ratios become important as the condition advances. Access to a swimming or hydrotherapy pool with appropriate changing facilities will be important.

The curriculum for boys with muscular dystrophy needs to adapt to the progression of the condition. Interventions could include maintaining skills and abilities while providing appropriate levels of support. It is not unusual for boys to have difficulties with basic literacy and numeracy skills, which are sometimes linked to variable concentration. Computers with appropriate adaptations can provide continued access to information. Independence skills and PSHE (personal, social and health education) are areas that require careful attention. PE needs modification to include these boys while compensating for weakness and poor coordination – for example, a light plastic cricket bat can be used when a wooden one is too heavy. Team games can be made inclusive by having runners (other children) or by allowing affected boys to be the scorer. Swimming is often encouraged as a physical activity that can be sustained long term and will help with maintaining muscle strength. Curriculum balance can become an issue when requirements of a physical preventative programme begin to impact on other subjects. An extended school day could provide more time.

Attention should be given to the provision of pastoral care. The self-esteem of boys can diminish with their loss of motor ability and the changing timetable. A positive and constructive attitude is required in an inevitably deteriorating situation. There may be questions from other pupils and adults in the school, while questions from affected boys themselves could indicate the need for counselling and/or the monitoring of mental health and emotional well-being.

Useful links
Duchenne Family Support Group
37a Highbury New Park
London N5 2EN
Tel: 0870 606 1604 (Family Helpline)
Tel: 0870 241 1857 (Office)
E-mail: dfsg@duchenne.demon.co.uk

Muscular Dystrophy Campaign
7–11 Prescott Place
London SW4 6BS
Tel: 020 7720 8055
E-mail: info@muscular-dystrophy.org

Dwarfism *see Achondroplasia*

Dysarthria

This is a general term for defective speaking, usually due to slurring or poor articulation. It is often seen in children with cerebellar, peripheral motor or muscular defects (see *Speech disorder*).

Dysarthrophonia

Problems with speech production originating in the brain or elsewhere in the central nervous system also affect voice production, nasality and breathing. It can lead to excessive hoarseness, a high-pitched voice or squeaky voice quality (see *Speech disorder*).

Dyscalculia

This is the term used when children's ability to understand and use mathematical concepts is significantly lower than might reasonably be expected. School-based *Interdisciplinary working* including the advice of an educational psychologist who has specialised in this work and specialist teachers is important. Effective links with parents can be very helpful. Good pastoral arrangements will provide support for these children and include opportunities to celebrate success and reinforce self-esteem.

Children with dyscalculia need help in organising and processing information related to numbers and mathematical concepts. It is important to communicate simply and clearly with a child when he or she is tackling mathematical problems. It is useful to try to convey the same idea or concept in a number of ways in order to find the most helpful way for that particular child: some children are very literal while others benefit from graphic explanations. The language of mathematics uses numbers, so any simple games and exercises that are number-based can be helpful. A successful strategy is to use the practical day-to-day activities that take place at home and at school to give the child something concrete on which to base their understanding. For example, have a child help with counting how many books or pencils are needed to be given out in a classroom, or be responsible for counting the dinner numbers.

Multisensory approaches to teaching have proved very successful for many children with dyscalculia; a frequently used approach is Visual, Auditory, Kinaesthetic and Tactile (VAKT). A child taking part in number activities will normally see, hear and say numbers; using a multisensory approach adds touch and movement. There are some excellent software packages that provide strong visual images with sound and the use of a touch-screen provides the kinaesthetic dimension. Pictures can be useful when mathematical problems are being described. If you are using pictures, get the child to 'draw' the process leading to the correct solution. Work a problem through repeating the stages carefully and get the child to repeat them back. Read the problem out loud and encourage the child to listen very carefully, as this builds on auditory skills. Produce work on worksheets that are uncluttered and do not contain too much visual information. In

young children the use of music poetry and rhythm can help with memorising facts or rules. Adapt the numeracy strategy creatively, ensuring that the basic principles are sensible and well ordered. Where accreditation and examination work is concerned, seek the necessary concessions – this usually requires a report from an educational psychologist.

Overall, children with dyscalculia will need ongoing attention to their learning and will respond best to praise and encouragement.

Useful links
The Dyscalculia Site
Earlstrees Court
Earlstrees Road
Corby NN17 4HH
Tel: 01536 399004
E-mail: firstandbest@thE-mail.co.uk
www.dyscalculia.org.uk

Dysfluency

Dysfluency occurs when there is a problem with producing a smooth flow of speech. It is more noticeable in the primary phase when a child is learning to express new, abstract concepts. Most children will become more fluent as they get older and their language skills improve. The timing of any intervention becomes a matter of judgement; it is very important to have open and frank communication with parents. Early intervention is generally more effective than waiting until the matter has become more complex to treat and manage. Serious concerns about a child's fluency will need a referral to a speech and language therapist who will be able to tell whether speech and language developments are similar to those of other children of the same age. Referrals can be more speedily made by parents through their own General Practitioner.

Working with children who are dysfluent can be time consuming. The advice in *Speech and language problems* will apply. It is vital to give a child confidence and support, so teachers and class-based staff need to avoid drawing attention to the problem by interrupting, criticising, completing sentences, correcting or looking pained or exasperated. It is good practice to listen closely and pay attention to what the child says rather than the way it is said. Use a slow rate in speech and pause frequently. A slow speaking rate provides a good model for a child and gives the child more time to understand and formulate thoughts. Provide a model of appropriate language by repeating back to a child what has been communicated. Provide opportunities for the child to talk to staff without distractions or competition from other pupils. Reduce pressure on the child to communicate, limit the number of questions asked and do not demand that the child make an immediate response. Through observations of different situations, build up an understanding of those times or places that increase or decrease fluent behaviour. Recognise that certain language factors can have an effect on fluency. For example, dysfluency can increase if a topic is unfamiliar and involves complex language, is difficult to understand, or refers to something that happened in the past. Recognise that certain environmental factors may have a negative effect on fluency, such as time pressure, arguing, fatigue, new situations,

unfamiliar listeners, competition to speak or excitement. It is unlikely that the curriculum should be significantly modified for children because they are dysfluent.

Useful links
The British Stammering Association
15 Old Ford Road
London E2 9PJ
Tel: 020 8983 1003
www.stammering.org/

The Michael Palin Centre for Stammering Children
Finsbury Health Centre
Pine Street
London EC1R 0LP
Tel: 020 7530 4238
E-mail: info@stammeringcentre.org
www.stammeringcentre.org/feedback/cont act.html

Dysglossia

Physical malformation of peripheral speech organs can present at birth or occur in later life (e.g. paralysis, harelip, cleft palate or jaw) (see *Speech disorder*).

Dysgraphia

Dysgraphia means difficulty with writing for no obvious reason. Children with dysgraphia might produce writing that is distorted or incorrect, make inappropriately sized and spaced letters, or write incorrect or mis-spelled words. They may have other learning disabilities, for example *Dyslexia*; however, they often have no social or other academic problems.

Children with dysgraphia will emerge as the demands for written work increase. The signs of dysgraphia include illegibility and inconsistency in text and layout. The mechanisms of writing can be unusual, such as pencil grip and body position, or over-laboured copy-writing; the child carefully watches his or her hand while writing, and in general has a level of written ability not as well developed as other communication skills. Where dysgraphia is recognised, a good diagnostic assessment, educational programme, curriculum planning and overall monitoring are essential to assist the child to progress with writing.

School-based *Interdisciplinary working,* including the advice of an educational psychologist who has specialised in this work and specialist teacher is important. Effective links with parents can be very helpful. Good pastoral arrangements will provide support for these children and include opportunities to celebrate success and reinforce self-esteem.

Teachers wanting to reduce the demand for written work will need to consider making more time for work to be done, reducing the amount to be produced, making the written tasks as simple as possible and allowing the pupil to use the means of writing that best suits them, such as a particular pencil or pen, word processor, or writing via speech recognition software, etc. The written component of lessons can be reduced by looking creatively at other means and media including oral reports and pictorial representations. Where a child's educational programme has recommendations and advice on how to teach handwriting, these should be applied sensitively and supportively. Where accreditation and examination work is concerned, seek the necessary concessions; this usually requires a report from an educational psychologist.

Overall children with dysgraphia will need ongoing attention to their learning and will respond best to praise and encouragement.

Dyslexia

Dyslexia means 'difficulty with words'. It is thought that children with dyslexia may have a difference in the part of the brain that deals with language and this affects the skills that are needed for learning to read, write and spell. Dyslexic children process information differently but, with a different approach, can learn effectively.

Children with dyslexia have their special educational needs met throughout the education service. There is much written, and there are differences of opinion, about what is dyslexia and how children with dyslexia should have their special educational needs met. It is beyond the scope of this book to address the differences of opinion. Labelling a child as dyslexic or as a classification within the subsets of dyslexia is not necessarily productive unless it results in strategies that are going to help the child learn.

Good diagnostic assessment, a carefully designed educational programme, effective curriculum planning and monitoring are essential to support children in making progress. School-based *Interdisciplinary working,* including the advice of an educational psychologist who has specialised in this work, specialist teachers and therapists is important. Effective links with parents can be very helpful. Good pastoral arrangements will provide support for these children and include opportunities to celebrate success and reinforce self-esteem.

As children with dyslexia experience problems with written language, access to the written elements of the curriculum will need attention. Some subjects rely heavily on written information; it is therefore very important for children with dyslexia at KS3+4 to have developed effective learning strategies or to have necessary support and means in place to provide them with good curriculum access. Where accreditation and examination work is concerned, seek the necessary concessions – this usually requires a report from an educational psychologist.

A structured programme addressing the child's needs is essential and is likely to be based on the teaching of phonological coding and include specific approaches to teaching spelling and handwriting. Multisensory approaches to teaching have proved very successful for many children with dyslexia; a frequently used approach is Visual, Auditory, Kinaesthetic, and Tactile (VAKT). A child reading will normally see hear and say words – using a multisensory approach adds touch, movement and the possibility of dividing words up into easy-to-learn parts. There are some excellent software packages providing strong visual images with sound and the use of a touch-screen provides the kinaesthetic dimension. The necessary time to work on a multisensory approach means spending more teaching time with the child. The structure and content of sessions recommended through the national literacy strategy can be most helpful and very supportive of those children with dyslexia.

Teachers and staff working with children with dyslexia will need to follow the specific advice of specialists carefully. It is important to use classroom practices that will support learning; for example, keep the child in reasonably close proximity to provide help, develop the child's oral strategies and find a way of focusing on those rather than written responses, encourage repeating back (auditory memory), take care with presentations, and take time to find which particular styles, fonts and colours of written material are easiest for the child to read. For some children it is helpful to use computers or word processors; some keyboards will suit more than others. Differentiate in short-term planning, particularly where there is additional classroom support. Handwriting can be assisted where cursive script is used as early as possible. It is important that staff have some understanding of how the day-to-day variability in performance can lead to frustration, which in turn might lead to poor behaviour. When setting homework, make sure that this is understood by the child before it is time to go home; it can be useful to establish a daily notebook or diary, as this can be used to note work covered in school and to confirm homework. This can also serve as a useful means of communicating between home and school. When marking work, do not correct everything, for example marking written work on content not spelling. If possible sit with the child when going through his or her work and take the opportunity to praise oral contributions.

Children with dyslexia will need ongoing attention to their learning and will respond best to praise and encouragement.

Useful links
The British Dyslexia Association
98 London Road
Reading RG1 5AU
Tel: 0118 966 2677
E-mail: admin@bda-dyslexia.demon.co.uk
www.bda-dyslexia.org.uk

The Dyslexia Institute
133 Gresham Road
Staines TW18 2AJ
Tel: 01784 417300
E-mail: staines@dyslexia-inst.org.uk
www.dyslexia-inst.org.uk

Dysphonia

Dysphonia is an abnormality in the quality of the speech sounds and language produced by the child. It can be caused by problems with control of breathing, the vocal cords or other muscles in the head and neck that help produce speech sounds.

Children with dysphonia can be educated in mainstream and special schools. School-based *Interdisciplinary working* involving a physiotherapist and a speech and language therapist might be necessary for some children, while community medical services will manage others. Effective links with parents and good pastoral arrangements will provide support for these children. Work on the relaxation of the muscles of the larynx is carried out through programmes designed by a speech and language therapist. Exercises can include laughter and singing – with young children it might be possible to include these in whole class activities; for older children it can be helpful to provide

withdrawal. It is unlikely that the curriculum should be modified for children because they have dysphonia.

Useful links
Dystonia Society
46/47 Britton Street
London EC1M 5UJ
Tel: 020 7490 5671
www.dystonia.org.uk/dystoniasocietyh.html

Dyspraxia

Dyspraxia predominantly affects the child's ability to attain increasingly complex motor skills. It is also known as clumsy child syndrome, developmental motor disability and minimal brain dysfunction. It is thought to affect around 1 in 20 children, and is more common in boys. The typical picture would be of a child with difficulty in dressing and undressing, reversing clothes, having difficulty in tying shoe laces or doing up zips or fastenings. They tend to fall more often than their peers and have difficulties in sports and PE due to poor coordination and delayed eye–hand skills. Sequencing tasks are difficult and memory and sense of time is consequently often poor. Many children also have relationship problems and might exhibit secondary behaviours to avoid tackling tasks that they find difficult. These problems can ultimately lead to substantial educational underachievement.

Children with dyspraxia can be educated in mainstream and special schools. School-based *Interdisciplinary working* involving a physiotherapist and an occupational therapist might be necessary for some children, while community medical services will manage others. Effective links with parents and good pastoral arrangements will provide support for these children.

Because children with dyspraxia have a developmental difficulty in the planning and sequencing of coordinated movement, they need frequent and regular attention in order to learn new skills. Teachers and learning support assistants need to have sensitive and careful working practices with children with dyspraxia. Staff need to work positively and enthusiastically, keeping lessons simple and being explicit about learning objectives. With well-coordinated programmes, children make progress. Regular individual support in the classroom will help in the shaping and exercising of motor skills, and assist in improving attention span, handwriting and organisation skills. Children with dyspraxia will benefit from extra sessions of all early learning activities because, until they have developed good gross motor skills, they will find fine motor activities difficult.

The involvement of an occupational therapist and a physiotherapist is important. They can be particularly helpful in advising on the right kind of seats and tables. Good seating and positioning aids learning. The child needs to be anchored with feet flat on the floor – it can be beneficial to have a seating wedge to transfer weight through the hips and to the feet. Tables are better at hip height and, for some children, an angle board can support an arm, providing added stability to the upper torso. Anchoring legs and arms to help stabilise the pelvis and shoulders helps the child to sit still. The seat and table need to be positioned so that the child can easily see the teacher. Therapists and specialist teachers are able to break tasks and skills down into separate components and then reassemble them into a sequence. There are a large number of 'off the shelf' sequential analyses for tasks and skills such as writing, throwing and catching balls, riding a bicycle, etc. Where a therapist's clinics take place outside the school day, it is a good idea to establish a communication book between school, therapist and home to share information and to provide a common approach to support the child.

The child with dyspraxia may try to avoid physical activities and in particular the coordinated skills of PE. Some children will develop sophisticated avoidance strategies when expected to do tasks that they find too difficult. More recently the approaches of *Conductive education* have been recognised as beneficial for children with dyspraxia where there is an emphasis on small group work, body awareness, concentration and problem solving.

Useful links

The Dyscovery Centre
4a Church Road
Whitchurch
Cardiff CF14 2DZ
Tel: 02920 628222
E-mail: dyscoverycentre@btclick.com
www.dyscovery.co.uk

Dyspraxia Foundation
8 West Alley
Hitchin SG5 1EG
Tel: 01462 454 986
E-mail: admin@dyspraxiafoundation.org.uk
www.emmbrook.demon.co.uk

E-mail:
madeleineportwood@ukonline.co.uk
**www.ukonline.co.uk/members/madeleine.p
ortwood/dysprax.htm**

Dystonic cerebral palsy *see* Cerebral palsy

E

Echolalia

Echolalia is the repetition or echoing of verbal utterances made by another person. There are two types of echolalia: immediate echolalia and delayed echolalia. Most children use echolalia to learn language. The majority of children babble in a rhythmic way, which is actually mimicking the cadence of adult language. Later, they copy sounds, words, and eventually phrases and sentences that they hear adults use in specific, repetitive contexts. Children who use echolalia have not fully made the transfer to an understanding of the component parts of language and so they continue to repeat back the chunks that they have heard and this may or may not be meaningful. The acquisition of language is not a clear-cut changeover from echolalia to spontaneous language but rather is a continuum, which reflects not just the choice of words but also the evolution of the way that the child thinks and looks at the world. Echolalia therefore also appears to be a 'normal' step in the child's language acquisition. Children with autism may use echolalia as a part of their repertoire of communication (see *Autism*).

Children with echolalia can be educated in mainstream and in special schools. Effective links with parents and good pastoral arrangements will provide support for these children. School-based *Interdisciplinary working* should involve a speech and language therapist and specialist language teachers as it is important to establish why the child is using echolalia. There are a small number of approaches used by therapists to help children with echolalia for example 'cues-pause-point' which is a picture system supporting the spoken word and verbal modelling. The latter is more easily included into the daily work of classrooms. It is unlikely that the curriculum should be modified for children because they have isolated echolalia.

Eczema

Eczema is caused by inflammation of the skin. Most children have allergic (atopic) eczema. The skin is red and itchy. Scratching may further damage the skin leading to infection and eventually thickening of the skin. Treatment is with creams to stop the skin from drying out (which is when it becomes itchy) and with steroid creams to damp down the inflammation of the skin. Most children outgrow their eczema.

Children with eczema are generally effectively treated in the community by their General Practitioner. Because this is a skin reaction to an irritant or an allergy, by the time children attend school they will know what to avoid in the school environment. The school will need to do all that is possible in order to provide an allergy or irritant free environment. In extreme cases school staff will need the advice of a dermatologist or specialist allergy nurse. It is unlikely that the curriculum should be modified for children because they have eczema.

Useful links
British Association of Dermatologists
19 Fitzroy Square

London W1T 6EH

Tel: 020 7383 0266

Fax: 020 7388 5263

E-mail: admin@bad.org.uk

www.skinhealth.co.uk/contact/index.htm

Eisenmenger's syndrome

Eisenmenger's syndrome is a complication of congenital heart disease caused by excessive blood flow through the lungs for prolonged periods. The result is that the blood vessels in the lungs (where the blood is enriched with oxygen) resist the flow of excessive blood and the heart works harder and harder to overcome this. Eventually the heart muscle cannot contract powerfully enough to pump the blood through the lungs and the child's blood becomes progressively less well oxygenated. The condition causes increasing blueness (cyanosis) and exercise limitation. The only effective treatment is heart–lung or lung transplantation (see *Congenital heart diseases*).

Elective mutism

Elective mutism means that children are able to speak but remain silent with certain people or in certain settings. It is common when a child joins a different school. Children with elective mutism can prove to be very challenging but with coordinated and careful working many improve with time. There are more girls than boys with elective mutism. Teachers and staff will need to work closely and effectively with parents, an educational psychologist as well as a speech

and language therapist in designing an approach to help – see *Interdisciplinary working*. Research and experience indicate that forcing children to speak is not helpful, that children are unlikely to 'grow out of it' and that approaches and interventions work better when they occur in the places where the child does not speak.

Plans and strategies are generally highly individualised and include the best ways of addressing the child's mutism. All those working with the child need to be aware of the difficulty and should maintain a positive approach to all utterances and know not to force the child to speak. Where possible emphasise activities that do not involve spoken language such as writing, reading, drawing or computer-based learning. If appropriate, look for other means of communication such as signs, symbols and pictures. Ensure that the child is subject to the same expectations as peers. Include the child in team games and assemblies, link the child with other children who may also be friends out of school, keep the child in the same groups for work in the classroom, see if favourite activities can be built into lessons and try to plan for work that depends on children collaborating in order to complete tasks and report back to the class. Establish regular short periods of withdrawal for language work with a small number of other children to provide opportunities for expression. Where possible use the child's friendships within class groupings. Programmes to address elective mutism need to be advanced very slowly using those people to whom the child will speak as much as possible. More than anything else praise sounds or words the child actually makes and use concrete reward systems. Overall children with elective mutism have a condition that will to some extent effect their education.

Useful links

http://easyweb.easynet.co.uk/simplepsych /mutism.html

SimplePsych is a psychology site.

Emotional and behavioural difficulties (EBD)

Children's values, understandings and behaviour are largely shaped by family, environment, early experiences, social mores and the ethos of the community in which they live. As children grow up, the influences of the school, peers and media become increasingly important. Children can have EBD because of a range of factors. It is beyond the scope of this book to cover all that is encompassed within the understanding of EBD. The spectrum of emotional and behavioural difficulties includes mild but persistent bad behaviour, anxieties that prevent learning and severe mental health disorders requiring segregation and highly specialised interventions. There is no doubt that behaviour in the classroom is one of the most important issues currently facing many schools and all that work in them.

Children with EBD have their educational needs met in mainstream and specialist settings. EBD are frequently related to other conditions and/or disorders. It is useful for all staff to have basic training and awareness of the range of conditions and factors that may impact on children's emotional well-being, including conditions such as *ADHD*, *Autism*, *Dyslexia* and *Dyspraxia*.

In all situations where pupils' self-esteem and emotional well-being are concerned, the school's arrangements for pastoral care, behaviour and discipline will be influential. Children and young people will need high-quality care and attention at key times in the school day. This means that the school must be organised to allow appropriately trained staff to have the flexibility to spend time with pupils when they need it.

Where pupils require an individualised approach to the management of their behaviour, it is important to devise an individual behaviour management plan with parents, the educational psychologist and other professionals. It is important for teachers and staff in schools to work effectively with staff from other teams and agencies including specialist behaviour support teachers, educational psychologists and therapists – see *Interdisciplinary working*. Good communication with supportive parents can be extremely effective.

In order to adequately support children with emotional and behavioural difficulties, a school needs the following:

- clarity and consistency for pupils, parents and staff
- a good and challenging curriculum that interests pupils, and
- effective leadership, where teachers and the wider staff team are valued and held in high esteem.

In the classroom it is important that all staff raise self-esteem whenever possible, praise children when they achieve, make sure that things work as they should, prepare for changes well in advance and plan well so that any unforeseen happenings can be easily overcome.

Sometimes a child's behaviour escalates and may reach a point where they or others will be hurt. In these situations physical intervention cannot be avoided. The use of positive handling requires skill, judgement and knowledge of non-harmful methods of control. Appropriate training that is relevant and fits within the culture and ethos of the setting concerned is required. In specialist settings it is necessary to ensure that all staff are trained in appropriate techniques for positive handling and that there is a well-coordinated and frequently revisited approach known and worked to by all members of staff. There are a number of approaches and packages available to schools including assertive discipline, positive behaviour reinforcement, circle of friends and nurture groups. Groups of schools can determine a common approach or an education authority might recommend a particular package.

The work of nurture groups can be very helpful in supporting children with significant EBD. Nurture grouping is based on attachment theory, where a teacher and assistant will work closely with a small group of children with emotional and behaviour problems that are preventing their learning. Teacher and assistant will model and promote positive behaviour and social skills in a safe, predictable nurturing environment. As children progress they are reintegrated into their classes. Schools operating nurture groups find that there are significant benefits for all their children as the principals of nurture are absorbed into pastoral systems. The successes of nurture groups are noted

in *Excellence for All Children: Meeting Special Educational Needs* (DfEE, 1997).

To support school improvements, the Qualifications and Curriculum Authority (QCA) have produced guidance on setting improvement targets for pupils' emotional and behavioural development. Behaviour criteria scales give schools the means of systematically 'measuring' behaviour and therefore setting targets for improvement. Special schools for pupils with EBD will already be using sophisticated measures for their pupils. The QCA scales will help in other settings by making it possible to set a baseline for a group of children against which progress can be measured. (*Supporting School Improvement Emotional and Behavioural Development.* Qualification and Curriculum Authority, 2001. Ref. QCA/01/717.)

There is an increasing recognition that a large group of children have emotional and behavioural difficulties because of mental disorder. Official figures recognise that 1 in 10 children between the ages of 5–15 years will have a mental health problem (*The Mental Health of Children and Adolescents in Great Britain.* Stationery Office, 1999. A summary download can be found at www.statistics.gov.uk/statbase/Product.asp?vlnk=3983&More=N.). This authoritative report provides important information and makes the case that EBD are linked to social factors such as social class and family functioning and that the channelling of these children into medical services makes little sense. There is a disturbingly high correspondence between special educational needs and mental disorder; similarly mental disorders are higher where there is social deprivation. The report argues strongly for more resources to be made available for schools to enable them to support children in mental distress. It is clearly stated that staff working in schools need to be trained to distinguish between the 1–2% of children who have organic problems such as hyperactivity and autistic spectrum disorders that can be helped medically and those with urgent emotional and social problems such as shyness, anxiety, depression and impulses to self-harm that need other social interventions.

Teachers and those working in schools come under increasing pressure to succeed with children and young people with EBD. It is obvious that they cannot change some things, for example parenting, housing, employment, substance abuse and crime. There is a view that a new perspective on behaviour and emotional well-being is required. Society needs to reconsider its approach to these troubling issues and reconfigure the role and relationships of schools and education within a society where no one input stands alone.

Useful links
Association of Workers for Children with Emotional and Behavioural Difficulties (AWCEBD)
Charlton Court
East Sutton
Maidstone ME17 3DQ
Tel: 01622 843104
Fax: 01622 844220
E-mail: awcebd@mistral.co.uk
www.awcebd.co.uk

British Institute of Learning Disabilities (BILD)
Wolverhampton Road
Kidderminster DY10 3PP
Tel: 01562 850251
E-mail: bild@bild.demon.co.uk
www.bild.demon.co.uk

National Association of Special Educational Needs (NASEN)
NASEN House
4/5 Amber Business Village
Amber Close
Amington
Tamworth B77 4RP
Tel: 01827 311500
E-mail: welcome@nasen.org.uk
www.nasen.org.uk

TEAM TEACH Ltd
32 Church Street
Warnham RH12 3QR
Tel: 01403 268928
E-mail: George@team-teach.co.uk
www.team-teach.co.uk

Encephalocele

Encephalocele is a congenital condition where either part of the brain, its coverings (meninges) or both, forms a fluid-filled cyst outside of the skull. There is an associated failure of the skull bones to close through which the cyst protrudes and increased pressure within the brain can result (raised intracranial pressure). It can usually be treated by surgical closure, and increased fluid pressure can be controlled with a *Ventriculoperitoneal shunt*. It can be associated with *Spina bifida*. There can be other abnormalities of the nervous system, such as blindness and learning difficulties.

Children with encephalocele can be educated in mainstream and in special schools some will need highly specialised provision (see *Physical disability* and *Visual impairment*). School-based *Interdisciplinary working* involving a physiotherapist, an occupational therapist and specialist teachers might be necessary for some children, while community medical services will manage others. Effective links with parents and good pastoral arrangements will provide support for these children. Children with encephalocele will need access to the same curriculum as their peers.

Useful links
Association for Spina Bifida and Hydrocephalus
42 Park Road
Peterborough PE1 2UQ
Tel: 01733 555988
E-mail: postmaster@asbah.org
www.asbah.org/

Endocarditis *see* Atrial septal defect (ASD); Patent ductus arteriosus

Enthesitis-related arthritis see Arthritis

Enuresis *see* Daytime wetting; Neuropathic bladder; Nocturnal enuresis;

Epidermolysis bullosa

Epidermolysis bullosa is a condition where the skin is extremely fragile and blisters following minimal trauma. Some children present shortly after birth while others are less severely affected. Children with this problem may also have abnormal nails and the blisters can become infected. Severely affected children can have mobility problems from joint contracture, and difficulties with dexterity because of fusion of the finger tips. Feeding can be a problem if there is scarring of the mouth (see *Microstomia*) and swallowing difficult if the gullet is also similarly scarred.

Children with epidermolysis bullosa can be educated in mainstream and special schools. The extent to which epidermolysis bullosa affects schooling depends on the medical interventions required should the child's skin be rubbed or damaged in any way. For some children pain management is important while others might experience long periods of restricted mobility and will need exercises designed by a physiotherapist. School-based *Interdisciplinary working* might be necessary for some children, while community medical services will manage others. Effective links with parents and good pastoral arrangements will provide support for these children. Some children can appear very different and classmates should be appropriately informed about epidermolysis bullosa and encouraged to be supportive and thereby avoid any adverse comments (see *Disfigurement and difference*).

Children with epidermolysis bullosa will need access to the same curriculum as their peers. They may present as underachievers because of frequent absence from school and have lower expectations made of them because of their physical and medical problems. Staff should be aware of the supportive things that they can do in the event of a problem. Some children will require specially made clothing or uniforms, as seams can rub and cause problems. Gloves may need to be worn and these can be problematic when the child is writing or for activities needing fine motor skills. Most children are knowledgeable about the ways to manage their treatment but may need support with some dressings. A school needs good systems of support and opportunities for children to catch up after absences following treatments. Children in the primary phase may need special attention, as they might not tell staff when there is discomfort or a problem with a dressing because they are engrossed in a particular activity or because they might prefer to avoid treatment. Special arrangements will probably be needed to provide access to some sporting activities; swimming is possible but advice may be necessary where skin has abraded. The safety measures for all pupils are generally sufficient. Overall children with epidermolysis bullosa have a chronic condition that can sometimes interfere with their education.

Useful links
British Association of Dermatologists
19 Fitzroy Square
London W1T 6EH
Tel: 020 7383 0266
Fax: 020 7388 5263
E-mail: admin@bad.org.uk
www.skinhealth.co.uk/contact/index.htm

DEBRA
DEBRA House
13 Wellington Business Park
Dukes Ride

Crowthorne RG45 6LS
Tel: 01344 771961
E-mail: debra.uk@btInternet.com
www.debra.org.uk

Epilepsy

Epilepsy is a condition where children have recurrent fits – these are also known as convulsions or seizures. A fit is caused by brain cells firing off in a chaotic and uncontrolled manner. The whole surface of the brain can be involved in this process causing a generalised seizure, whereas when just one part of the brain is involved then the child has a partial seizure. Generalised seizures can cause the child to lose consciousness, fall to the ground and jerk – this is known as 'grand mal'. In other generalised seizures the child might blank out for a few seconds, become still and have odd facial movements such as flickering of the eyelids, known as 'petit mal' or absence epilepsy. Children who have absence epilepsy can look as though they are 'daydreaming' during an episode. This can cause confusion when children who daydream because they are bored or unengaged in a task are suspected of having this form of epilepsy. Children who daydream are usually interruptible and can be brought back on task. Children who are having episodes of absence epilepsy cannot be interrupted. Some children have seizures that cause episodes of strange behaviour or might pick at clothing or exhibit other repeated activities. These children have complex partial seizures, where only part of the brain is involved and the child's consciousness is altered, but not lost. Most fits are short lived, but in some children fits can be prolonged. Longer fits can potentially be dangerous, particularly those where the fits prevent the child breathing effectively. This is known as status epilepticus, and requires urgent treatment. Children in school who are known to have episodes of status epilepticus will need special plans for their treatment; this may involve the administration of rectal diazepam (Valium) and calling an ambulance. This method of giving medication is necessary, as an unconscious child cannot safely swallow medicines by mouth. Certain activities can pose increased risks for children with epilepsy in school. For this reason climbing high on PE apparatus, unsupervised swimming and cycling on open roads are often prohibited.

In most cases epilepsy can be treated with anticonvulsant drugs. Occasionally more than one drug is needed. Sometimes other treatments such as surgery, special diets or other techniques are required. Children with learning difficulties are more likely to have epilepsy. Epilepsy itself can cause difficulties with learning; either directly because fits interfere with the child's ability to access the curriculum, or indirectly because epilepsy can cause difficulties with learning. Some of the medications used to treat epilepsy can cause cognitive side effects themselves, which further complicates this issue. Children with epilepsy might have other neurological or developmental/learning difficulties that can affect their access to the curriculum. Children can feel isolated and unconfident in themselves and face overprotectiveness from their families. This in turn might affect their transition from dependent chil-

dren to independent adults.

Children with epilepsy have their educational needs met in mainstream and special schools. Their education can be disrupted in some way either by the absences or seizures that they have or by the side effects of medication. Effective *Interdisciplinary working* including good communication networks can be very important particularly at times when medical management strategies are changing. Children with epilepsy will have a useful understanding of how they are affected; they might for example experience a warning (aura) before having a seizure.

It is important for all staff involved in working with children with epilepsy to have appropriate training and to be familiar with the particular aspects of an individual child's epilepsy. They need to be able to recognise seizures and calmly know what to do about them. It is very important for staff teams to develop good observation skills in order to record epileptic episodes for parents and the extended professional teams. Good information based on observation helps formulate management strategies that evolve for a child over time. Observations noting the triggers, the length and description of the seizure or absence and what happens afterwards are very helpful. A child's intellectual, physical or emotional well-being can be changed by some anticonvulsion medications.

Attention should be given to the school environment to make sure that there are minimal hazards. In the event of children having a seizure and then needing to rest or sleep afterwards, suitable arrangements should be made with parents. Some children may sleep or rest at school and then return to lessons; for others it may be preferable for them to sleep or rest at home.

The curriculum may need varieties of adaptation as some children may be learning more slowly than others because their medication has an adverse effect on their ability to learn, while other children might miss large parts of the taught day because of seizures or absences. There tends to be little that can be done about effects of medication on learning. Where children miss parts of the school day, then all efforts need to be made to compensate at other times such as extended days, home tuition and creative use of homework.

The school's pastoral systems and ethos are very important indeed, as children with epilepsy need to be provided with emotional, psychological and social support. They need to feel confident about their epilepsy and about themselves. All other children in the school need to be educated so that they are not alarmed when witnessing seizures or absences, and they need to be encouraged to grow up having positive and helpful attitudes towards epilepsy.

In general children with epilepsy should not be unnecessarily restricted, although judgements of this kind need to be made with parents. For example, it would not be sensible for a child who experiences regular seizures to be asked to climb high apparatus. For children known to have regular seizures it is advisable for them to be accompanied one-to-one when swimming. It is safe for children with epilepsy to swim provided that lifesavers are informed and know how to support a child having a seizure in the water. Going on school and residential trips requires simple preplanning and preparation. Staff may be asked to administer medication or to supervise a child self-medicating. It is important that this function is carried out within the clear advice provided by the local education authority and/or school governors, school health service and professional association or trades union.

Useful links
British Epilepsy Association
New Anstey House
Gateway Drive
Yeadon
Leeds LS19 7XY
Tel: 0808 800 5050
E-mail: helpline@bea.org.uk
www.epilepsy.org.uk

DfES Publications Centre
PO Box 5050
Sudbury CO10 6ZQ
Tel: 0845 6022260
www.dfes.gov.uk/medical/

Supporting Pupils with Medical Needs – a Good Practice Guide *is a document to help schools draw up policies on managing medication in schools, and to put in place effective management systems to support individual pupils with medical needs. This can be downloaded from DfES website.*

Erythema multiforme

Erythema multiforme is a skin rash. It occurs after certain infections or in response to certain drugs. It is usually short lived. The rash itself is not infectious, although it can look quite dramatic. When the lips, mouth and other mucous membranes are also involved the condition is known as *Stevens–Johnson syndrome.*

Children with erythema multiforme can be educated in mainstream and special schools. The extent to which erythema multiforme affects schooling depends on the medical interventions required. Most children will have their condition managed by community medical services. Effective links with parents and good pastoral arrangements will provide support for these children. Some children can appear very different – classmates should be appropriately informed about erythema multiforme and encouraged to be supportive and avoid any unnecessary comments (see *Disfigurement and difference*).

The curriculum will not need to be modified for children because they have erythema multiforme.

Useful links

British Association of Dermatologists
19 Fitzroy Square
London W1T 6EH
Tel: 020 7383 0266
Fax: 020 7388 5263
E-mail: admin@bad.org.uk
www.skinhealth.co.uk/contact/index.htm

The Rare Disorders Alliance
www.cafamily.org.uk/rda-ukhtml

Four limb cerebral palsy *see* Cerebral palsy

Fractures

Fractures of the bones in otherwise healthy children occur as the result of trauma. This can be due to falls, road traffic accidents or sometimes, physical abuse. When a bone breaks there is pain, swelling and loss of function in the affected limb. There can also be redness, bruising or bleeding. Treatment is aimed at getting the broken bones to heal up. This might require a splint, plaster, operation or a combination of these approaches. Depending on the site of the fracture, mobility, self-care and manipulation can be affected for some weeks.

Children with fractures can be educated in mainstream and special schools. The extent to which fractures affect schooling depends on the medical interventions required. Most children will have their condition managed by community medical services. Effective links with parents and good pastoral arrangements will provide support for these children. Although there can be some temporary disruption and absence, it is unlikely that the curriculum should be modified for children because they have fractures of the bones.

Fragile X

Fragile X is a condition affecting the development of boys, although girls can be carriers of the condition and can also be affected. Boys with this condition are usually quite large for their age, but often have low muscle tone and delayed motor, self-care, social and language development. Their communication skills are often delayed, and they can behave in a similar manner to autistic children. Children have learning difficulties that vary from mild to severe. These difficulties often become more apparent as the child gets older.

Children with fragile X are affected in different ways and have their educational needs met in mainstream and special schools. Children can show any the following characteristic behaviours: impulsivity, inattention, hyperactivity and mimicry. They might exhibit anxiety in social settings and like routines and repetitive behaviours.

Speech and language are almost always affected. It is not unusual for children to skip rapidly from topic to topic while in conversation and to repeat the last word or phrase spoken to them (a condition known as *Echolalia*). The advice and guidance of a speech and language therapist following a communication assessment can prove helpful (see *Interdisciplinary working*).

It is helpful to minimise additional auditory and visual distractions when communicating. Keep the amount of information transmitted to manageable chunks as some children find it more difficult to make sense of large quantities of information. Learning objectives are better packaged into simple sets or sequences that last no more than 10 or 15 minutes with frequent opportunities for repetition. Some curriculum differentiation will almost certainly be necessary, and some children might require additional classroom support.

Research and experience has shown that children with fragile X can find mathematics particularly difficult where conceptual learning is involved. It is preferable to keep to the simplest and most direct teaching methods possible through visually based materials and approaches. Similarly multisensory approaches to teaching have proved very successful; a frequently used approach is Visual, Auditory, Kinaesthetic, and Tactile (VAKT). A child adding numbers together will normally see, hear and say the values; using a multisensory approach adds touch and movement. There are some excellent software packages that provide strong visual images with sound and with use of a touch-screen providing the kinaesthetic dimension. School-based *Interdisciplinary working* including the advice of specialist teachers might be useful in developing a multisensory programme.

Reading and spelling can be relative strengths, with some children achieving 'average' performance. Learning a sight vocabulary is usually significantly easier than learning phonics; therefore the literacy strategy may need adapting accordingly. Paired reading can be successful. Handwriting can present problems, so the use of word processing can be helpful.

Classrooms need to be as calm and uncomplicated as possible, with relatively few distractions. It is generally better to work from a position behind the child to reduce the need for eye contact. Keep to familiar and consistent classroom routines and keep the child informed of impending changes. The use of a personal work area or work-station can be beneficial. Hyperactivity in

children with fragile X tends to decrease with age, but attention difficulties and impulsivity can remain problematic for many adolescents. Some children do present teachers with management problems in the following ways: by getting up on impulse, meandering around the classroom, reacting vigorously and inappropriately to events around them or by appearing uncooperative at times. Many children will benefit from a carefully designed behaviour management plan; in these situations it is sensible to seek the advice of an educational psychologist.

Useful links
Fragile X Society
53 Winchelsea Lane
Hastings TN35 4LG
Tel: 01424 813147
E-mail: lesleywalker@fragilex.k-web.co.uk
www.fragilex.org.uk

Friedreich's ataxia

Friedreich's ataxia causes unsteadiness when the child moves. Speech is also eventually affected causing slurring. The spine also often becomes deformed (scoliosis) and the heart muscle can be affected. The illness can result in a reduced lifespan from the heart and spinal problems. Vision can be affected through *Nystagmus*, and some individuals suffer hearing problems and *Diabetes mellitus*.

Affected children face difficulty with mobility, communication and manipulation. They also have to cope with the progressive nature of the condition.

Children with Friedreich's ataxia can be educated in mainstream and special schools.

They need care, attention and consideration as the effects of the condition progress. School-based *Interdisciplinary working* will be necessary including the advice of specialist teachers, speech and language therapists and possibly an educational psychologist. Class teams should develop detailed assessment, recording and reporting strategies in order to support the medical assessments that mark the progress of the condition. Good pastoral arrangements should be in place to support the child and to provide support to peers.

Attention will need to be given to those aspects of the school's environment that can prove difficult as the child experiences increasing physical difficulty (see *Physical disability* and *Dyspraxia*). Adaptations will be needed to PE and games to give the child similar experiences to their peers. Swimming is a good alternative to some of the more specifically demanding sporting activities.

Some children experience slurred speech and need opportunities to work on exercises designed by speech and language therapists and/or specialist teachers (see *Speech disorder*).

If hearing and vision are affected, then the curriculum should be suitably modified by appropriately qualified and trained staff. Children with Friedreich's ataxia have a condition that will inevitably significantly affect their education.

Useful links
Ataxia
10 Winchester House
Kennington Park
Cranmer Road
London SW9 6EJ
Tel: 020 7582 1444 (Office)
E-mail: office@ataxia.org.uk
www.ataxia.org.uk

G

Gastrostomy *see* Artificial feeding

Glaucoma

Glaucoma is a condition that occurs when the pressure inside the eye becomes abnormally high. There may be resulting loss of vision, which can, if not detected in time, become severe and permanent. In young children, it is sometimes known as bupthalmos. The condition can affect both eyes. Children might have enlarged eyes, pain and intolerance to light. Treatment usually involves surgery. The ways in which glaucoma can affect the eye will vary. For further advice see *Visual impairment*.

Children with glaucoma can be educated in mainstream and special schools. School-based *Interdisciplinary working* including the advice of a specialist teacher for visual impairment might be necessary for some children, while community medical services will manage others. Effective links with parents and good pastoral arrangements will provide support for these children.

A child may be able to see an object one day and be unable to do so the next. These children may also have better peripheral than central vision and thus look at objects out of the side of their eye. They can have visual field losses that are not symmetrical (one eye might be worse than the other). Children with glaucoma experience problems with specific types of visual tasks. They have difficulty with figure-ground (seeing an object instead of the background), and with complex visual displays. Spatial confusion is common; for example being unable to locate their chair even though they can see it. The curriculum should be modified for children because they have glaucoma.

Useful links
Hands and Eyes
A USA specialist teacher maintains this useful online newsletter for teachers and caregivers of visually impaired students and their friends. It includes art, cooking and manipulative activities that visually impaired students can do individually or in small groups. It is for teachers and support staff in need of ideas for classroom activities and is particularly useful for pupils with multiple impairments such as developmental disability and motor impairment.
www.home.earthlink.net/~vharris/

RNIB Education Information Services
224 Great Portland Street
London W1N 6AA
Tel: 020 7388 1266
E-mail: webmaster@rnib.org.uk
www.rnib.org.uk
RNIB's curriculum information service offers information and advice to all professionals supporting a visually impaired child in mainstream or special schools.
www.rnib.org.uk/curriculum/
RNIB's accessing technology pages provide information about applications of technology in employment, at study and in leisure.
www.rnib.org.uk/technology/

V.I. Guide
This site contains information on many topics relating to parenting and teaching a child with visual impairments.
www.viguide.com/

Globoid cell leukodystrophy *see* **Leukodystrophies**
Glomerulonephritis

Glomerulonephritis is inflammation of the kidneys. The condition sometimes follows a throat infection and sometimes is due to other infections or immune problems. The child might have raised blood pressure that requires treatment or in other cases may require medication to reduce the inflammation in the kidneys. Children lose blood or protein in the urine. In some cases the inflammation can cause ongoing damage to the kidneys that results ultimately in renal failure (see *Renal dialysis*).

Children with glomerulonephritis can be educated in mainstream and special schools. School-based *Interdisciplinary working* might be necessary for some children; others will have their condition managed by community medical services. Effective links with parents and good pastoral arrangements will provide the child with support.

Some children with glomerulonephritis will need special arrangements for when they experience symptoms. Symptoms include fatigue, nausea and vomiting, shortness of breath, disturbed vision and swelling of the face, hands, feet and ankles. In these circumstances you will need to judge whether the child can continue working at an activity. Overall children with glomerulonephritis have a condition that could temporarily affect their capacity to access the curriculum.

Useful links
National Kidney Federation
6 Stanley Street
Worksop S81 7HX
Tel: 0845 601 0209
E-mail: helpline@kidney.org.uk
www.kidney.org.uk

Nephronline
E-mail: info@nephronline.org
www.nephronline.org/

Glue ear see Otitis media

Goitre *see* Hypothyroidism

Grommets

Grommets are tiny tubes that are surgically inserted through the eardrum to allow air into the middle ear. This allows the pressure on either side of the eardrum to equalise and, in turn, lets the drum function more normally and hence improves hearing. Most are designed to come out over time. It is a treatment for conductive hearing problems that occur when a child is affected by glue ear. The surgeon who performed the operation will give the parents advice about swimming (or its avoidance), which should be passed onto the school.

Children with grommets can be educated in mainstream and special schools. School-based *Interdisciplinary working* involving specialist teachers might be necessary for some children, while others will have their grommets managed by community medical services. Effective links with parents and good pastoral arrangements will provide support for these children. Children with grommets will need different types of attention depending on how successfully they function. It is not unusual for the grommets to fall out rapidly and they do not always work effectively. Dependant on the extent of hearing loss, the advice found under *Hearing impairment* will apply. Hearing tests and medicals take place regularly in school. Ideally these should not adversely affect educational provision.

Growth hormone

A deficiency in this hormone causes short stature, as the hormone is required for the growth of the bones and tissues. Some children can be treated with replacements of growth hormone by injection (see *Short stature*). Occasionally excessive growth hormone is secreted from the pituitary gland causing tall stature or abnormally fast growth.

Useful links
Growth Hormone Deficiency Support Group
c/o Child Growth Foundation
2 Mightfield Avenue
Chiswick
London W4 1PW
Tel: 020 8995 0257

Growth hormone deficiency *see* Growth hormone

Guillain–Barré syndrome *see* Transverse myelitis

H

Haematuria

Haematuria is the passage of blood in the urine. It may be obvious and visible (macroscopic haematuria) or only detectable on special testing (microscopic haematuria). It can occur during *Urinary tract infections*, following trauma, in *Glomerulonephritis*, in children who develop kidney stones, or in those with bleeding problems.

Children with haematuria will have their educational needs met in mainstream and special schools. Most children will have their condition monitored and treated by community medical services. Effective links with parents and good pastoral arrangements will provide the child with support. It is unlikely that the curriculum will need to be modified for children because they have haematuria.

Useful links
Nephronline
E-mail: info@nephronline.org
www.nephronline.org/

Haemodialysis *see* Renal dialysis

Haemophilia

Haemophilia is caused by a lack of clotting factors in the blood, which are required to produce blood clots; the bloodstream normally produces these when a haemorrhage occurs. It mainly affects males and is carried by females. Boys with this problem can bruise easily and excessively. Trauma can cause obvious bleeding or bruising (bleeding into the skin). Bleeding into joints can occur and can show itself as a painful or swollen joint. There can also be redness, localised heat and loss of normal function of the joint; for instance the child may limp if the knee is affected. Internal blood loss is rare, although bleeding into the muscles is more common. Treatment is by replacing the missing clotting factor by an injection into the vein. Older children can be taught to treat themselves, as early treatment is important to reduce the chances of long-term disability.

Children with haemophilia can be educated in mainstream and special schools. The extent to which haemophilia affects schooling depends on the medical interventions required should the child get knocked or hurt in any way. School-based *Interdisciplinary working* might be necessary for some children; others will have their condition managed by community medical services.

Children with haemophilia will need access to the same curriculum as their peers. All staff should be aware of the particular things to do in the event of a bleed or a knock. Most children are knowledgeable about the way their disorder affects them and with support will deal with problems well. Good systems of communicating between home and school are necessary. When children do have an emergency, then it is helpful to have effective arrangements to get to hospital quickly or the place of treatment, with any necessary consents. Parents or carers should be contacted as soon as possible and children should not go home alone.

Children needing frequent absence from school and time-consuming treatments following bleeding episodes can lead to staff having low expectations of them and school friendships will be disrupted. It is important to explore all possible ways of supporting children who are regularly absent and to provide a range of ways to help them catch up with work; this becomes very important where children are mid-syllabus for externally accredited examinations.

Following a bleeding episode activity should be resumed gradually. As each bleeding episode can differ, it is helpful to ask parents if any changes need to be made to the guidance. Children in the primary phase may need special attention, as they tend not to tell staff when they know they are bleeding because they are engrossed in a particular activity or because they might prefer to avoid treatment. The advice of medical professionals will probably be needed to ensure that exercises, activities and games in PE are appropriate, as it is advisable to avoid all contact sports.

Children with haemophilia need to take gentle exercise – it is therefore important to develop other interests such as music, photography, modelling, craftwork, woodwork and metal work. The safety measures for all students around school are appropriate and are generally sufficient. Overall, children with haemophilia have a chronic, variable condition that sometimes can interfere with their education.

Useful links
Haemophilia Society
3rd Floor Chesterfield House
385 Euston Road
London NW1 3AU
Tel: 0800 018 6068
E-mail: info@haemophilia.org.uk
www.haemophilia.org.uk

Head injury

Head injury can result from road traffic accidents and falls, but can also result (particularly in babies) from non-accidental injuries following, for example, forceful shaking. The injuries depend on the type and magnitude of the event. The skull can be fractured and the fracture might press down onto the brain causing damage (depressed skull fracture). There may be bleeding under the skull that causes a build-up of pressure on the brain (extradural haemorrhage or subdural haematoma). There may be bleeding within the brain or direct damage to the substance of the brain. Treatment is usually undertaken urgently and consists of helping the child with their breathing and other vital functions. Although many children recover, many are left with residual impairments that can be lifelong. These depend upon the age and degree of development of the child and severity of the injury but broadly have educational implications similar to *Cerebral palsy, Epilepsy, Hydrocephalus, Visual impairment, Hearing impairment* and emotional and behavioural problems, including violence to themselves and others. The effects can be temporary or permanent and affect the subsequent development of the child into adulthood. These difficulties have the most concrete implications for the child at school.

Children with head injuries can be educated in mainstream and special schools.

The extent to which this condition affects schooling depends on the consequences of the damage. School-based *Interdisciplinary working* involving therapists might be necessary for some children, while others will have their condition managed based on community medical services. Effective links with parents and good pastoral arrangements will provide support for these children.

Children with head injuries will need access to the same curriculum as their peers. Educational programmes for these children will need to take account of specific impairment or disability. Suitable modifications to the environment and the curriculum are likely.

Useful links
Children's Head Injury Trust
Radcliffe Infirmary
Woodstock Road
Oxford OX2 6HE
Tel: 01865 224786
E-mail: enquiries@chit.demon.co.uk
http://glaxocentre.merseyside.org/chit.html

Head lice

Head lice (pediculosis) is a very common problem in schools. The infestation spreads quite easily amongst young children who spend much of the time at school in close proximity to one another. The term 'nits' is used to describe the egg cases that adhere to the hair follicles. Treatment with shampoo toxic to the lice is often recommended, although other techniques, such as repeated applications of shampoo and conditioner, followed by careful grooming with a fine-

toothed comb ('bug busting'), are also recommended by some. Re-infestation is common. Affected children usually only complain of itchiness of the head and neck.

When children get head lice, treatments are usually carried out by parents/carers following the advice provided by school health teams. A school generally needs to work alongside health colleagues to promote awareness, eradicate the stigma, identify infestations and teach children good healthcare habits. In some situations children and families will need support and counselling.

The curriculum will not need to be modified for children because they have head lice.

Useful links
British Association of Dermatologists
19 Fitzroy Square
London W1T 6EH
Tel: 020 7383 0266
Fax: 020 7388 5263
E-mail: admin@bad.org.uk
www.skinhealth.co.uk/contact/index.htm

Community Hygiene Concern
Manor Gardens Centre
6–9 Manor Gardens
London N7 6LA
Tel: 020 7686 4321
E-mail: bugbusters2k@yahoo.co.uk
www.chc.org

Hearing aids

Some children will need hearing aids in order to receive speech. Hearing aids work on the same basic system, a microphone arrangement that amplifies sound through an earphone. The user generally is able to exercise some control over the volume and tone of the output. As technology progresses the sophistication and refinements of these devices improve. There are individual aids such as 'behind the ear' aids, group aids (where children are physically connected to one piece of equipment), loop induction systems, individual radio systems and infrared systems.

It is not unusual for children in the primary phase to show some resistance to wearing an aid, particularly if it does not 'look good'. These days there are some appealing bright and cheerful aids. Whatever system is used, a good strategy is to develop the child's independence rapidly in their management of the aid. The younger child will need more assistance and support but by secondary school it would be reasonable to expect independence other than in extreme circumstances.

Most conventional hearing aids work best within a 2–3 metre radius, as beyond that, other background noise will interfere. It is important to be aware of this range for direct instruction and group activities. No aid will allow a child to hear exactly as would be possible if he or she had no hearing loss. The aid is designed to amplify accurately all sounds – it is therefore reasonable to expect the aid to work within its limitations without having to go to any elaborate lengths. If the aid does not do what the child needs, then parents will need to request something else. It is sensible to have spare batteries and leads available in school. Batteries last longer if stored in a cool place or the fridge. It is sometimes useful to know the arrangements for loans or repairs should there be a malfunction.

Although hearing aids are one of the most common forms of amplification technology used, an FM radio device might be recommended. Here the teacher wears a microphone, which sends the speech directly to the ears of the child through headphones or loudspeakers. This ensures that regardless of where the child is within the room, they will hear the teacher's voice as if only 6 inches away. A lapel or throat microphone is generally used by the teacher, as this amplifies the voice and not the background noises created by other children or elsewhere in the environment. Teachers and staff using microphones need to avoid banging them on jewellery or buttons and to speak in a normal tone of voice. Teachers and children participating in assemblies will need to wear a microphone. Similarly the position of an omnidirectional microphone needs to be considered for open discussion sessions and small group work. An FM system will usually transmit for a distance of approximately 45–50 metres. The child will need to have a clear view of the speaker's mouth to receive all of the information. The gymnasium and school trips can be difficult hearing environments.

Useful links
Royal National Institute for Deaf People
19–23 Featherstone Street
London EC1Y 8SL
Tel: 020 7296 8000
E-mail: informationline@rnid.org.uk
www.rnid.org.uk/index.htm

Hearing impairment

Deafness or hearing difficulties can arise from many causes and conditions. It can affect one or both ears. The level of deafness is variable from child to child and by condition. The definition and severity are defined by the loudness (measured in decibels) of sound exhibited to a person before they are able to detect it. People whose hearing ability is within the normal range can detect sounds louder than approximately 0–20 dB (a whisper). Mild impairment is present when the intensity of the sounds required is between 21 and 40 dB (level of normal background noise at home). Moderate deafness occurs when the loss is between 40 and 70 dB (conversational voice). Severe loss occurs at between 70 to 90 dB (cocktail party noise level) while profound loss occurs when intensities beyond 90 dB (discotheque or shouting level) are required. The hearing loss can be temporary (as with a cold), fluctuating (for example with glue ear) or progressive. The point at which the hearing difficulties first emerge is also important. For example, severe hearing difficulties in prelingual children may prevent the development of inner language as well as normal expressive speech.

Children with hearing impairments can be educated in mainstream and special schools. School-based *Interdisciplinary working* involving specialist teachers, audiologists and audio technicians might be necessary for some children, while community medical services will manage others. Effective links with parents and good pastoral arrangements will provide support for these children.

Children who are deaf or have a hearing impairment that is a significant barrier to learning will require additional specialist support. Inexperienced staff working in schools will require specialist training, advice and support. Many children with a hearing loss will need a hearing aid. Hearing aids work on the same basic system with a microphone arrangement that amplifies sound through an earphone. The user generally is able to exercise some control over the volume and tone of the output. As technology progresses the sophistication and refinements of these devices improve. There are individual aids such as 'behind the ear' aids, group aids (where children are physically connected), loop induction systems, individual radio systems and infrared systems. For more detailed information see *Hearing aids*.

Children with hearing impairments will hear better in places with good acoustic properties. For all children and particularly for children with hearing impairments, it is sensible to attend to those things that will improve the quality of sound to support hearing and listening. Classrooms and other spaces in schools tend to have poor acoustics. There is a considerable difference in the sound quality in rooms that have hard surfaces and that in rooms with carpets and wall hangings. It is helpful to reduce reverberation and noise by applying sound absorbing materials to as many hard surfaces as possible. Attention needs to be given to lighting as it is vital that the hearing-impaired child can see the teacher so that they can 'read' lips or see signs clearly. Lip reading and facial expression is an important element of receiving spoken language for all children with hearing impairments. It can be very useful to ask an experienced teacher of hearing-impaired children to carry out an assessment of the school and recommend measures to improve acoustics.

There is a long-standing controversy among some professionals working with children who are deaf or have hearing impairments. Some professionals believe that signing should be the prime method of communication; others believe that children should learn to speak and to lip read and not be taught manual signing. There are some professionals who oppose the use of manual signing in any form on the basis that the hearing-impaired child will have to live in a world of hearing and speaking people and must therefore learn to understand spoken language and learn to speak. The debate within education has been long and complex and will continue into the future. Most children with hearing impairments will develop good oral communication supported by lip reading and be able to express themselves using spoken language. Where there is uncertainty over oracy or signing for a child, then the decision needs to be made with parents based on unbiased factual information. Where children with hearing impairment need significant levels of support with their communication, both oral and signed, then they are likely to be taught in specialist settings. There will always be some children who are profoundly deaf who will have to use manual signing. It is preferable for these children to be taught signed English rather than British Sign Language (BSL) as it supports the learning of reading and writing. Although BSL is used throughout the UK and uses the vocabulary of English, it has a grammar of its own and may follow a different syntax to spoken English. It is very important for children using BSL and learning to read and write to have specialist advice and support.

In most classrooms children with hearing impairments will be developing spoken language alongside their peers. It is likely that the speech of the hearing-impaired child will vary from the speech used by classmates, although this will be specifically determined by the type and degree of the hearing impairment. It will be important to work closely with specialist teachers and speech and language therapist to support the child to help produce the most intelligible speech possible and to develop speech sounds and speech patterns. Hearing-impaired children can have difficulties controlling aspects of voice production, and it is particularly important that these skills are carefully and specifically taught from the earliest possible age. It is very important to encourage the child to talk as much as possible and not to stop the child to 'correct' speech. On those occasions where speech is not understood, then staff need to calmly and carefully ask for it to be repeated once only. Care, consistency and a clear focus is needed by all working with hearing-impaired children to help them produce the best speech possible.

Lessons and the teaching arrangements for children with hearing impairments should be suitably differentiated according to the severity of the hearing impairment. Attention will clearly need to be given to all aspects of communication including comprehension and expression. Very young children in play settings will be physically active and are likely to need more frequent attention to the hearing aids they use.

Patience and determination with the very young child with hearing impairment to help put in place strategies for learning and compensating will bring very real benefits in later years. Staff working with very young children with hearing impairments need to learn as much as possible about the child in order to make best use of preferred learning styles, attention span and specific interests. All staff need to encourage early involvement with books and stories. Take care that the literacy strategy is not dogmatically applied; for example, work on phonics might need to be extended for the child working on sound and voice production, but might not be so appropriate to the child who is using BSL.

Valuing the hearing-impaired child's achievements in all lessons helps to raise their self-esteem, which in turn is important in developing their confidence in communicating with others. At all times, staff need to include the hearing-impaired child in questions and conversations. It is helpful to develop simple strategies such as before asking a question, say the child's name, and get his or her attention.

- Always face the child (and the class).
- When speaking, talk clearly and naturally.
- Use body language and explicit non-verbal communication consistently.
- Avoid excessive head movements. Use the board and other supporting media while noting the preferred media of the hearing-impaired child.
- Ensure that when you are using TV or video captions or subtitling systems work easily.
- Write down words and graphically illustrate ideas, always making sure that homework and other assignments are given and are available in a written form.
- Do not use oral tests for any formal purposes.
- Learn how to unobtrusively check for understanding and learning.
- Give the hearing-impaired child preferential seating if possible with the light behind so that they can see speaking adults well. This also helps with lip reading and non-verbal communications through eye contact, facial expressions and gesture.
- Shut the door of the classroom to cut down on background noise and distractions.
- Where listening is particularly important such as in stories and music, pay particular attention to helping children concentrate.

Children with impaired hearing can get tired easily from the continuous strain of keeping up. Make allowances by providing opportunities to take breaks or to move on to tasks with a different focus.

Where children are using signing to communicate, it is important to remember to speak and sign simultaneously. To make signing fun, use signs that the child will know; similarly make use of their interests and experiences. Encourage accuracy – crisp signing is better for all. Watch the signing child carefully and adapt lessons to ensure they are included. Other children without hearing impairments will learn and use sign language, and this can only be beneficial.

In small group settings it is important to

encourage the hearing-impaired child to face the pupil/s speaking and to encourage peers not to 'chatter' but to speak in turn. A hearing-impaired child will not immediately know where sound or speech is coming from, so it can be useful to develop a visual cueing system to identify the current speaker. Before introducing a new topic for class discussion it is probably sensible to enlist the help of parents in familiarisation of new vocabulary or of the class tasks or discussion topics planned. When questioning the whole class, always repeat the correct answer once given. In some sessions and settings it is helpful to make sure that children with hearing impairments are grouped or paired with those children most likely to support and care. This can be important when they are on the playing field or in places with poor acoustic qualities such as gym halls or swimming pools.

It is important for staff to keep good systematic records of children's progress in expressive and receptive communication; these will assist in deciding how the communication programme should develop; it also provides parents with information about progress.

Useful links
deafPLUS
Prospect Hall
12 College Walk
Selly Oak
Birmingham B29 6LE
Tel: 0121 415 2080
E-mail: info@deafplus.org
www.deafplus.org

The National Deaf Children's Society
15 Dufferin Street
London EC1Y 8UR
Tel: 020 7490 8656
Helpline: 020 7250 0123
E-mail: fundraising@ndcs.org.uk
www.ncds.org.uk

RNID
19–23 Featherstone Street
London EC1Y 8SL
Tel: 0808 808 123
E-mail: informationline@rnid.org.uk
www.rnid.org.uk

Heart block

Heart block is a rare congenital condition where the normal conduction of impulses through the heart that cause coordinated contraction of the heart muscle is disturbed. The condition can be treated by placing fine wires into the heart and stimulating the heart (pacing) with a specially implanted electrical device (pacemaker) (see *Congenital heart diseases*).

Hemiplegia *see* Cerebral palsy

Henoch–Schönlein purpura

Henoch–Schönlein purpura is a bruise-like rash that can affect children, often following a viral infection. Affected children can also suffer from joint and abdominal pains. The kidneys are often involved and blood is sometimes detected in the urine. In most children the problem is short lived; very occasionally there can be long-term consequences if the kidneys continue to be affected. The child and their rash are not infectious.

Children with Henoch–Schönlein purpura can be educated in mainstream schools. The extent to which Henoch–Schönlein purpura affects schooling depends on the ways in which the symptoms present themselves and the consequent medical interventions required. School-based *Interdisciplinary working* might be necessary for some children, while community medical services will manage others. Effective links with parents and good pastoral arrangements will provide support for these children.

Children with Henoch–Schönlein purpura will need access to the same curriculum as their peers. Staff should be aware of the supportive things they can do in the event of a problem. Overall, children with Henoch–Schönlein purpura have a temporary condition that can sometimes interfere with their education.

Useful links
British Association of Dermatologists
19 Fitzroy Square
London W1T 6EH
Tel: 020 7383 0266
Fax: 020 7388 5263
E-mail: admin@bad.org.uk
www.skinhealth.co.uk/contact/index.htm

Hepatitis

Hepatitis is the term given to infections that cause inflammation of the liver, leading to reduced functioning. For example, the breakdown of the yellow pigment, bilirubin, can be inhibited producing a build-up in the skin and in the whites of the eyes. This is known as jaundice. Hepatitis A can cause outbreaks at schools as it can be spread by mouth. Hepatitis B, C and D are not spread orally but can affect children from certain high-risk groups. Children with hepatitis B are not at risk of infecting others at school during normal daily activities, but sensible precautions should be taken if you have to deal with body fluids (blood, faeces, urine, vomit) from infected children. In practice precautions including the wearing of disposable gloves should be used when or if coming into contact with body fluids.

Children with hepatitis can be educated in mainstream and special schools. The extent to which hepatitis affects schooling depends on the symptoms and the time taken for children to get well. Some children may experience fatigue for several months following the illness. A school needs good systems of support and opportunities for children to catch up with school work after absences. Generally children will have their condition managed by community medical services. Effective links with parents and good pastoral arrangements will provide support for these children. It is unlikely that the curriculum should be modified for children because they have hepatitis.

Useful links
British Liver Trust
Central House
Central Avenue
Ipswich IP3 9QG
Tel: 01473 276326
E-mail: info@britishlivertrust.org.uk
www.britishlivertrust.org.uk

Children's Liver Disease Foundation
36 Great Charles Street
Birmingham B3 3JY
Tel: 0121 212 3839
E-mail: info@childliverdisease.org
www.childliverdisease.org

Hirschsprung's disease

Hirschsprung's disease occurs when a part of the lower bowel develops without the nerves that are required to make the bowel propel faeces along normally. The result can be very troublesome *Constipation* requiring special surgery to treat it effectively.

Children with Hirschsprung's disease can be educated in mainstream and special schools. The extent to which Hirschsprung's disease affects schooling depends on how children learn to manage their condition. School-based *Interdisciplinary working* might be necessary for some children; others will have their condition managed by community medical services. Effective links with parents and good pastoral arrangements will provide support for these children.

Some children with Hirschsprung's disease will need special arrangements to enable them to get to toilets when they need to (see *Physical disability*). Overall these children have a condition that may need attention during the school day but should not be a reason to modify the curriculum.

Useful links
Gut Motility Disorders Support Network
7 Walden Road
Sewards End
Saffron Walden CB10 2LE

Tel: 01799 520580
E-mail: help@gmdnet.org.uk

HIV *see* Human immunodeficiency virus

Human immunodeficiency virus (HIV)

Most children with HIV contract the disease from their mothers during pregnancy, delivery or breastfeeding. Children born to mothers with HIV do not necessarily contract the disease, although rates of transmission in developing countries are much higher than those in Europe. Children who are affected might go on to develop immune deficiency. In severe case this leads to developmental delay or progressive learning difficulties, pneumonia, failure to thrive and possibly to malignancy. The child can also suffer from unusual infections and diarrhoea. More mildly affected children have enlarged lymph glands and swelling of the parotid gland at the angle of the jaw causing facial swelling. Children will be on treatment regimens to halt progression from HIV infection to AIDS. The risk of catching HIV from an infected child is small and the normal precautions that should be taken with every child are all that is required. Most children with HIV will have parents with HIV.

Children with HIV can be educated in mainstream and special schools. Some children experience long and frequent periods of illness together with complex courses of treatment. Frequent absence from school for time-consuming treatments can lead to staff having low expectations of children's achievements and school friendships will be disrupted. It is important to explore all possible ways of supporting children who are regularly absent and to provide a range of ways to help them catch up with work; this becomes very important where children are mid-syllabus for externally accredited examinations.

Members of the same family might be infected so careful *Interdisciplinary working* will be necessary with a community health team including specialist workers. The school's pastoral systems should be effective in supporting children in all aspects of their life. The local education authority and health authority will issue very specific guidance on how schools should manage the circumstances of having children with HIV in school.

Useful links
Barnardo's Positive Options
William Morris Hall
6 Somers Road
Walthamstow
London E17 6RX
Tel: 020 8520 6625

National AIDS Helpline
Tel: 0800 567 123
Free, confidential 24-hour advice service for HIV/AIDS.

Positively Women
347–349 City Road
London EC1V 1LR
Tel: 020 7713 0222
E-mail: info@positivelywomen.org.uk
www.positivelywomen.org.uk

The Terrence Higgins Trust Lighthouse
52–54 Grays Inn Road
London WC1X 8JU
Tel: 020 7242 1010
E-mail: info@tht.org.uk
www.tht.org.uk

Hunter disease *see* Mucopolysaccharidosis

Hurler disease *see* Mucopolysaccharidosis

Hydrocephalus

Hydrocephalus is a condition where there is excessive cerebrospinal fluid – this presses on the brain matter thereby causing damage and potential disability. Untreated, it can cause drowsiness, vomiting, blindness and eventually coma and death. It can be caused when there is a blockage in the normal drainage systems that help circulate the cerebrospinal fluid around the brain and spinal cord. It is often treated surgically by the insertion of a *Ventriculoperitoneal shunt*.

Children with hydrocephalus can be educated in mainstream and special schools. The extent to which this condition affects schooling depends on the extent of any damage and the medical interventions required. Some children will need frequent and regular visits to hospital and will need exercises designed by a physiotherapist. School-based *Interdisciplinary working* involving a physiotherapist and an occupational therapist might be necessary for some children, while others will have their condition managed by community medical services.

Effective links with parents and good pastoral arrangements will provide support for these children.

Children with hydrocephalus will need access to the same curriculum as their peers (see *Spina bifida* and *Physical disability*). Frequent absence from school and time-consuming treatments can lead to low expectations. It is important to explore all possible ways of supporting children who are regularly absent and to provide a range of ways to help them catch up with work. This becomes very important where children are absent mid-syllabus for externally accredited examinations. Some children will spend long periods in wheelchairs, therefore access to classrooms and other school buildings needs to be good. Work requiring fine motor skills should be adapted as some children cannot hold pencils easily and may need specialised keyboard access. The advice of medical professionals might be needed to ensure that exercises, activities and games in PE are appropriate.

Useful links
Association for Spina Bifida and Hydrocephalus
42 Park Road
Peterborough PE1 2UQ
Tel: 01733 555988
E-mail: postmaster@asbah.org
www.asbah.org/

Hyperacusis

Children with hyperacusis have a heightened sensitivity to ordinary sounds. Everyday noises such as industrial machinery, heater blowers, sirens or something falling to the floor can seem unbearably loud. Children with *Autism* and *Williams syndrome* can also have hyperacusis.

Children with hyperacusis can be educated in mainstream and special schools. School-based *Interdisciplinary working* might be necessary for some children, while community medical services will manage others. Effective links with parents and good pastoral arrangements will provide support for these children. It is sensible to attend to those things that will improve the quality of sound to support hearing and listening. Classrooms and other spaces in schools tend to have poor acoustics. There is a considerable difference in the sound quality in rooms that have hard surfaces and the sound quality in rooms with carpets and wall hangings. It is helpful to reduce reverberation and noise by applying sound absorbing materials to as many hard surfaces as possible. It can be very useful to ask an experienced teacher of hearing-impaired children to carry out an assessment of the school and recommend measures to improve acoustics. It is unlikely that the curriculum should be modified for children because they have hyperacusis.

Hypercholesterolaemia

Hypercholesterolaemia is a metabolic condition that runs in families. Affected children have very high levels of cholesterol in the blood and are at high risk of suffering from cardiovascular disease in early adulthood. Some children may have a skin rash produced by deposits of the cholesterol in the skin, but generally there are no symptoms in childhood. Treatment is with diet and cholesterol-lowering drugs.

Children with hypercholesterolaemia can be educated in mainstream and special schools. The extent to which hypercholesterolaemia affects schooling depends on the medical interventions required. School-based *Interdisciplinary working* might be necessary for some children, while most will have their condition managed by community medical services. Effective links with parents and good pastoral arrangements will provide support for these children.

Children with hypercholesterolaemia will need access to the same curriculum as their peers. Special arrangements will probably be needed to provide access to physically demanding sporting activities. The safety measures for all pupils are generally sufficient. It is unlikely that the curriculum should be modified for children because they have hypercholesterolaemia.

Useful links
Family Heart Association
7 North Road
Maidenhead SL6 1PE
Tel: 01628 628638
E-mail: fh@familyheart.org
www.familyheart.org

Hypermetropia *see* Refractive error

Hyperthyroidism

Hyperthyroidism occurs when the thyroid gland is overactive and produces excessive amount of the thyroid hormone, thyroxine.

Affected children can grow abnormally quickly, have difficulties with learning and behaviour and they might be anxious. They can suffer from diarrhoea, a fast heart rate and eye problems. The condition is treatable with medicines by mouth, although sometimes surgery is required.

Children with hyperthyroidism can be educated in mainstream and special schools. The educational arrangements for children with this condition will vary widely between individuals. The large majority of children have the condition effectively treated by community medical services and will not require any special attention. Effective links with parents and good pastoral arrangements will provide support for these children.

Useful links
British Thyroid Foundation
PO Box 97
Clifford
Wetherby LS23 6XD

Hypertonia *see* Cerebral palsy

Hypoadrenalism *see* (Cushing's syndrome)

Hypoparathyroidism

Hypoparathyroidism is seen in some children who suffer from a defect of chromosome 22. These children also can have heart problems and *Immune deficiency* (DiGeorge syndrome). The hormone deficiency affects bone growth and calcium levels. Pseudohypoparathyroidism occurs when the child is insensitive to the effects of the parathyroid hormone. These children often have obesity, short fourth fingers and suffer from nodules under the skin. They often have learning difficulties. See also *Hypothyroidism*.

Children with hypoparathyroidism can be educated in mainstream and special schools. School-based *Interdisciplinary working* might be necessary for some children, while community medical services will manage others. Effective links with parents and good pastoral arrangements will provide support for these children. Children with lack of immunity can be regularly absent from school. A school needs good systems of support and opportunities for children to catch up after periods of absence. Children needing frequent absence from school and time-consuming treatments can lead to staff having low expectations of them and school friendships will be disrupted. It is important to explore all possible ways of supporting children who are absent for long periods and to provide a range of ways to help them catch up with work; this becomes very important where children are mid-syllabus for externally accredited examinations.

Children with hypoparathyroidism will need access to a suitably modified curriculum. The advice of medical professionals might be needed to ensure that exercises, activities and games in PE are appropriate.

Useful links
Max Appeal
Lansdowne House
13 Meriden Avenue
Stourbridge DY8 4QN
Tel: 01384 821227
E-mail: maxappeal@cableinet.co.uk
www.maxappeal.org

Hypoplastic left heart

Hypoplastic left heart occurs when the left collecting (atrium) and pumping (ventricle) chambers are underdeveloped. It coexists with a *Patent ductus arteriosus* and *Coarctation of the aorta*. This causes very serious illness in very young babies and operative approaches to treatment still have only limited success. See also *Congenital heart diseases*.

Hypospadias

Hypospadias is a condition where the tube that takes urine from the bladder emerges on the underside of the penis, rather than at the end. It can cause some continence difficulties and is usually treated surgically.

Boys with hypospadias can be educated in mainstream and special schools. School-based *Interdisciplinary working* might be necessary for some children, although most will have their condition managed by community medical services and it will not adversely affect schooling. Effective links with parents and good pastoral arrangements will provide support for these children. It is unlikely that the curriculum should be modified for boys because they have hypospadias.

Useful links
Hypospadias Support Group
20 Barnack Close
Padgate
Warrington WA1 4JH
Tel: 01925 496510
E-mail: clarkejn@aol.com
www.hypospadias.co.uk

Hypothyroidism

Hypothyroidism is caused by an underactive thyroid gland not producing enough of the thyroid hormone, thyroxine. This can cause developmental difficulties in very young children as well as a failure to thrive. In older children the deficiency might show itself as a child who starts to experience learning difficulty. Affected children can also have problems with weight gain, constipation, slower growth and dry skin. They can also have a lump in the front of the neck (goitre). Treatment is with replacement hormone, which can be given by mouth.

Children with hypothyroidism can be educated in mainstream and special schools. The educational arrangements for children with this condition will vary widely between individuals. The large majority of children have the condition effectively treated by community medical services and will not require any special attention. Some children will show intolerance to cold and tiredness. Effective links with parents and good pastoral arrangements will provide support for these children.

Useful links
British Thyroid Foundation
PO Box 97
Clifford
Wetherby LS23 6XD

Hypotonia

Hypotonia literally means low muscle tone. While many children can be affected by low muscle tone because of *Cerebral palsy* or other known diseases affecting the brain, nerve or muscle, others exhibit low muscle tone (often during early childhood) without a recognised cause. Many children with learning difficulties also have low muscle tone. This can also produce hyperextensible ('double') joints, frequent falls and delayed motor development.

Children with hypotonia can be educated in mainstream and special schools. The extent to which this condition affects schooling depends on the degree of low muscle tone and children's mobility. Some children will need exercises designed by a physiotherapist. School-based *Interdisciplinary working* involving a physiotherapist and an occupational therapist might be necessary for some children, while community medical services will manage others. Effective links with parents and good pastoral arrangements will provide support for these children.

For the child with low muscle tone, most difficulties are with mobility, fine motor activity and coordination. Attendant self-care difficulties can also be present. The advice about the school environment, curriculum and resources found under *Physical disability* will apply.

Useful links
UK Congenital Hypotonia
Flat 1, Frognal Court
158 Finchley Road
London NW3 5HL
Tel: 01462 454986
E-mail: tash@lacobrown.freeserve.co.uk
http://freespace.virgin.net/bch.hypotonia/

I

Ichthyosis

Ichthyosis is the presence of scaly skin seen in children born with congenital ichthyosis and related conditions. The skin appears in large scales and is itchy. Treatment is with creams to prevent the scales from drying out (it is this that causes the itching) and can also involve wrappings to prevent drying and reduce scratching. Children may have to contend with applying creams many times a day and also put up with the smell caused by bacteria growing in the abnormal skin. If the hands are severely affected , the child could have problems with dexterity.

Children with ichthyosis can be educated in mainstream and special schools. The extent to which ichthyosis affects schooling depends on the medical interventions required. For some children pain management is important, others can experience long periods of restricted mobility and will need exercises designed by a physiotherapist. School-based *Interdisciplinary working* might be necessary for some children, while community medical services will manage others. Effective links with parents and good pastoral arrangements will provide support for these children. Some children may appear very different – classmates should be appropriately informed about ichthyosis and are encouraged to be supportive and to avoid any unnecessary comments (see *Disfigurement and difference*).

Children with ichthyosis will need access to the same curriculum as their peers. Staff should be aware of the supportive things they can do in the event of a problem. Most children are knowledgeable about the ways to manage their treatment but may need support with some dressings. Some children experience long and frequent periods of absence for some treatments. Frequent absence from school for time-consuming treatments can lead to staff having low expectations of children's achievements and school friendships will be disrupted. It is important to explore all possible ways of supporting children who are regularly absent and to provide a range of ways to help them catch up with work; this becomes very important where children are mid-syllabus for externally accredited examinations.

Children in the primary phase may need special attention, as they might not tell staff when there is discomfort or a problem with a dressing because they are engrossed in a particular activity or because they might prefer to avoid treatment. Special arrangements will probably be needed to provide access to some sporting activities – swimming is possible but advice might be necessary where skin requires hydration treatment with moisturisers. The safety measures for all pupils are generally sufficient. Overall children with ichthyosis have a chronic condition that sometimes can interfere with their education.

Useful links
British Association of Dermatologists
19 Fitzroy Square
London W1T 6EH
Tel: 020 7383 0266
Fax: 020 7388 5263
E-mail: admin@bad.org.uk
www.skinhealth.co.uk/contact/index.htm

Ichthyosis Support Group
16 Cambridge Court
Cambridge Avenue
London NW6 5AB
Tel: 020 7461 9034
E-mail: ISG@ichthyosis.co.uk

Immature behaviour *see* Emotional and behavioural difficulties

Immune deficiencies

Immune deficiencies make the child more prone to infections, harder for them to shake them off, or liable to catch infections that other children would not normally catch. Children are either born with these problems, or they can be caused by some medical treatments such as chemotherapy for leukaemia or they sometimes follow infections. Treatment can be with low dose daily antibiotics (prophylaxis), full courses of antibiotics during infections, intravenous immune protein injections and, in some specific disorders, bone marrow transplant. Affected children are usually at risk of catching infections from other children rather than posing an infective risk to others.

Some children with immune deficiencies can be educated in mainstream, hospital and special schools; others can be significantly affected and be educated at home or in highly specialised environments. School-based *Interdisciplinary working* involving specialists might be necessary for some children, while others will have their condition managed by hospital or community medical services. Effective links with parents and good pastoral arrangements will provide support for these children. Children with immune deficiencies will need access to the same curriculum as their peers.

Useful links
Primary Immunodeficiency Association
Alliance House
12 Caxton Street
London SW1H 0QS
Tel: 020 7976 7640
E-mail: info@pia.org.uk
www.pia.org.uk

Impetigo

Impetigo is the name given to crusting infected skin sores. It is usually seen on the face and can be spread by the child touching, scratching or picking at the infected spots. Treatment is with antibiotics.

Many children will get impetigo. They are usually not permitted to be at school while they are infected as it is so contagious. Normal basic hygiene should be observed. Good communication between home and school is helpful while treatment is ongoing. When there is an outbreak in school, it is useful to get the support of the school nurse to provide good information to children and their families and to assist in making decisions about when the children are no longer infectious and can return to school. The curriculum will not need to be modified for children because they have impetigo.

Useful links
British Association of Dermatologists
19 Fitzroy Square

London W1T 6EH
Tel: 020 7383 0266
Fax: 020 7388 5263
E-mail: admin@bad.org.uk
www.skinhealth.co.uk/contact/index.htm

Inborn errors of metabolism

Inborn errors of metabolism are conditions where a specific chemical or set of chemicals (enzymes) required to use or to break down nutrients are missing. This omission causes a build-up of by-products from incomplete metabolism or a failure to produce essential substances for the body to use. These can lead to developmental, learning, behavioural or physical problems. Some inborn errors can cause severe bouts of illness that can threaten the child's life or development. Others cause a gradual build-up of toxins that produce a continuing deterioration in the child's functioning, development and learning. Some inborn errors cause jaundice and liver problems, while yet others produce epilepsy, developmental delay and learning difficulty; other systems can also be affected. Treatment is by avoiding foods that would normally be dealt with by the missing enzymes or by avoiding situations that require the missing enzyme to be active.

Children with inborn errors of metabolism can be educated in mainstream and special schools. School-based *Interdisciplinary working* involving specialist medical staff might be necessary for some children, while community medical services will manage others. Effective links with parents and good pastoral arrangements will provide support for these children. The educational arrange-ments for children with this condition will vary widely between individuals. A modified curriculum will be required for most children; for others, where there is progressive physical and cognitive disability, a highly differentiated curriculum with high levels of individual attention is needed. See also *Epilepsy* and *Physical disability*.

Useful links
Climb
The Quadrangle
Crewe Hall
Weston Road
Crewe CW2 6UR
Tel: 0870 770 0326
E-mail: info@climb.org.uk
www.climb.org.uk

Intoeing

Intoeing is also sometimes known as pigeon toes. The feet appear to turn inwards and can seemingly contribute to falls. It is caused by the slight inward twist of the tibia (shank bone) and sometimes the femur (thigh bone) in the child. Usually as the child ages, the bones straighten out and the problem gets better on its own. Very occasionally, in severe cases where the feet do not straighten, surgery is sometimes required to bring the feet into line.

Children with intoeing have their educational needs met in all schools. The advice about the school environment in *Physical disability* will apply. The curriculum should not need to be modified for children because they have intoeing; however, some children will be absent from school while receiving treatment.

Useful links
STEPS
Lymm Court
11 Eagle Brow
Lymm WA13 0LP
Tel: 01925 757525
E-mail: info@steps-charity.org.uk
www.steps-charity.org.uk

Irritable hip

Irritable hip causes temporary mobility problems by limiting movement at one or both hip joints. It is most often seen in young children and occurs with, or shortly after, a viral infection. It causes pain and limitation of movement around the hip joint. The condition is usually self-limiting and gets better without any specific treatment. Occasionally the difficulties recur and the condition can be confused with infections of the joint (septic arthritis – *see Osteomyelitis*).

Children with irritable hip can be educated in mainstream and special schools. School-based *Interdisciplinary working* involving a physiotherapist and an occupational therapist might be necessary for some children, while community medical services will manage others. Effective links with parents and good pastoral arrangements will provide support for these children.

The advice about the school environment found under *Physical disability* will apply. It is unlikely that the curriculum should be modified for children because they have an irritable hip.

Useful links
STEPS
Lymm Court
11 Eagle Brow
Lymm WA13 0LP
Tel: 01925 757525
E-mail: info@steps-charity.org.uk
www.steps-charity.org.uk

J

Jaundice *see* **Hepatitis**

Juvenile arthritis *see* **Arthritis**

K

Kearns–Sayre syndrome *see* Mitochondrial cytopathies

Keratitis

Keratitis is the name given to inflammation of the transparent central part of the eye, the cornea. It causes redness and pain and is due to bacterial or viral infections, and sometimes trauma (for instance, a scratch). Treatment can be with antibiotic drops or ointments, as well as patching of the eye. The condition is usually temporary, but can occasionally lead to serious visual problems.

Children with this condition can experience intense pain, discomfort and temporarily impaired vision; they may be intolerant to bright light (photophobia).

As the pain can be severe in keratitis, it is important to have good pastoral arrangements to provide children with appropriate support. Some children may experience permanent damage to their sight (see the advice in *Visual impairment*). Generally it is unlikely that the curriculum should be modified for children because they have keratitis.

Useful links
Hands and Eyes
A USA specialist teacher maintains this useful online newsletter for teachers and caregivers of visually impaired students and their friends. It includes art, cooking and manipulative activities that visually impaired students can do individually or in small groups. It is for teachers and support staff in need of ideas for classroom activities and is particularly useful for pupils with multiple impairments such as developmental disability and motor impairment.*
www.home.earthlink.net/~vharris/

RNIB Education Information Services
224 Great Portland Street
London W1N 6AA
Tel: 020 7388 1266
E-mail: webmaster@rnib.org.uk
www.rnib.org.uk
RNIB's curriculum information service offers information and advice to all professionals supporting a visually impaired child in mainstream or special schools.
www.rnib.org.uk/curriculum/
RNIB's accessing technology pages provide information about applications of technology in employment, at study and in leisure.
www.rnib.org.uk/technology/

V.I. Guide
This site contains information on many topics relating to parenting and teaching a child with visual impairments.
www.viguide.com/

Klinefelter syndrome

Klinefelter syndrome is caused in males by having an extra X (female) chromosome present. This often leads to children being relatively tall, but infertile in adult life as the testes do not develop normally. Some affected children also present in childhood with developmental problems or learning difficulties. These difficulties often revolve around processing visiospatial information (coordination) and with speech.

Boys with Klinefelter syndrome will need care and attention particularly while going through puberty. The advice and support of an appropriately trained counsellor will be important. The school's pastoral systems will need to provide support in all areas especially where physical differences are obvious. It is unlikely that the curriculum should be modified for boys because they have Klinefelter syndrome; however, some do experience some communication difficulties, especially with expressive language and others show low self-esteem that can lead to frustration and poor behaviour.

Useful links
Klinefelter Syndrome Association
56 Little Yeldham Road
Little Yeldham
Halstead CO9 4QT
Tel: 01787 237460
E-mail: p.dutton@ksa-uk.co.uk
www.ksa-uk.co.uk

Knee pain

Knee pain is very common in children and is thought to be caused in otherwise healthy children because of pressure on the knee joint. Discomfort can be treated with painkillers where appropriate.

Children with knee pain can be educated in mainstream and special schools. The extent to which this condition affects schooling depends on the medical advice. Some children experience periods of restricted mobility and will need exercises designed by a physiotherapist. School-based *Interdisciplinary working* involving physiotherapist might be necessary for some children, while most will have their condition managed by community medical services. Effective links with parents and good pastoral arrangements will provide support for these children.

Children with knee pain will need access to the same curriculum as their peers. The advice of medical professionals might be needed to ensure that exercises, activities and games in PE are appropriate.

Krabbe disease *see* Leukodystrophies

L

Labyrinthitis

Labyrinthitis is inflammation of the part of the inner ear concerned with maintaining balance. It is usually caused by a virus and leads to unsteadiness, falling and often nausea and vomiting. It is usually only a short-lived illness and gets better on its own. Children with labyrinthitis can experience sudden onset of *Vertigo* (a sensation of spinning or rotation) that can be severe enough to cause nausea or vomiting. The vertigo can come and go over periods of time. Children may also experience hearing loss, which is usually temporary. Advice found under *Hearing impairment* will apply.

Children with labyrinthitis can be educated in mainstream and special schools. Temporary school-based *Interdisciplinary working* might be necessary for some children, while community medical services will manage others. Effective links with parents and good pastoral arrangements will provide support for these children.

It is useful to have a whole school approach to supporting the child with labyrinthitis. Work with peers will be necessary so that they understand the condition and do not over-react to situations. A withdrawal room can be useful, as it will minimise interruptions to lessons. Some children will be affected more in specific circumstances – these can be physical, social or emotional, and it is sensible to find out about these in order to provide the best learning arrangements and to create safe and secure situations. It is unlikely that the curriculum should be modified for children because they have labyrinthitis.

Landau–Kleffner syndrome

Landau–Kleffner syndrome is a particular (and rare) form of childhood epilepsy that affects the understanding and use of language in a child who has previously developed normal linguistic skills. Fits may not be particularly prominent. The loss of language leads to communication and behavioural difficulties and the child might behave in an autistic fashion (see *Autism*). Diagnosis can require specialised brainwave (electroencephalogram – EEG) recordings and treatment is with antiepileptic medication. Some children are left with long-term problems and neurosurgical treatment is sometimes considered when there is a poor response to drugs.

Children with Landau–Kleffner syndrome can be educated in mainstream and special schools. The extent to which this condition affects schooling depends on the skills that children lose. School-based *Interdisciplinary working* involving medical specialists, a speech and language therapist and an educational psychologist will be necessary for most children while community medical services will manage others. Effective links with parents and good pastoral arrangements will be needed to provide the child with support (see *Epilepsy* and *Speech and language problems*).

Useful links
Friends of Landau–Kleffner Syndrome
3 Stone Buildings (Ground Floor)

Lincoln's Inn
London WC2A 3XL
Tel: 0870 847 0707
E-mail: RAHantusch@compuserve.com
www.bobjanet.demon.co.uk/lks

Leber's optic atrophy *see* Mitochondrial cytopathies

Leigh's disease *see* Mitochondrial cytopathies

Leukaemia

Leukaemia is a cancer of the white blood cells. Affected children can present with tiredness, anaemia, infections, and abnormal bruising and bone pain. Treatment is now largely successful at curing the disease, but the regimen is intensive and some parts of the treatment can cause immune deficiency, hair loss and, later on, difficulties in learning. Treatment often has an impact on the emotional and psychological well-being of the child and family.

Children with leukaemia can be educated in mainstream, special and hospital schools. School-based *Interdisciplinary working* might be necessary for some children while many will have their condition managed by hospital and community medical services. Effective links with parents and good pastoral arrangements will provide support for these children. Leukaemia might mean some children experience long and frequent periods of illness together with complex courses of treatment. Frequent absence from school for time-consuming treatments can lead to staff having low expectations of children's achievements and school friendships will be disrupted. It is important to explore all possible ways of supporting children who are regularly absent and to provide a range of ways to help them catch up with work; this becomes very important where children are mid-syllabus for externally accredited examinations.

Side effects of treatment need sensitive management. Children with leukaemia will need access to the same curriculum as their peers, although they can present as underachievers because of absence from school.

Useful links
CancerBACUP
3 Bath Place
Rivington Street
London EC2A 3JR
Tel: 020 7696 9003
E-mail: info@cancerbacup.org
www.cancerbacup.org.uk

Cancer Care Society
11 The Cornmarket
Romsey SO51 8GB
Tel: 01794 830300
E-mail: info@cancercaresoc.org
cancercaresoc.org

Cancerlink
Macmillan Cancer Relief
89 Albert Embankment
London SE1 7UQ
Tel: 0808 808 0000 or 020 7840 7840
E-mail: cancerlink@cancerlink.org.uk
www.cancerlink.org

CLIC
Abbey Wood

Bristol BS34 7JU
Tel: 0117 311 2600
E-mail: clic@charity.demon.co.uk
www.clic.uk.com

EDWARD'S TRUST
Edward House
St Mary's Row
Birmingham B4 6NY
Tel: 0121 237 5656

Leukaemia CARE Society
2 Shrubbery Avenue
Worcester WR1 1QH
Tel: 01905 330003
E-mail: leukaemia.care@ukonline.co.uk
www.leukaemiacare.org

Leukodystrophies

Leukodystrophies are a rare set of conditions that cause gradual loss of skills, increasing levels of disability, and increasing dependency as damage to the brain and nervous system progresses. These cause increased tone in the limbs, visual impairment and damage to the nerves to the limbs. Epilepsy and cognitive decline also occur. Adrenoleukodystrophy affects boys and is sometimes further complicated by problems with the functioning of the adrenal gland. A similar condition can affect both sexes in early (metachromatic leukodystrophy) and late (Krabbe disease or globoid cell leukodystrophy) childhood. This condition received popular attention in the 1993 film *Lorenzo's Oil*.

Children with leukodystrophy can initially have their educational needs met in main-stream schools; inevitably the progress of the condition will mean that they need very special care and a highly differentiated education. Children are likely to experience behavioural changes, declining memory, loss of emotional control and dementia. Other symptoms might include muscle weakness, difficulties with hearing, speech and vision. The rate of deterioration varies in each child and the curriculum will increasingly need highly specialised input from experienced and trained staff (see *Physical disability, Visual impairment, Hearing impairment*). The educational programme will need to include the maintenance of skills and providing the same curriculum entitlements of all children. As time goes by school-based *Interdisciplinary working* involving therapists will become necessary. The school will need to have excellent pastoral arrangements giving the children and their family high levels of support and counselling.

Children with leukodystrophies have a condition that will significantly affect their education.

Useful links
ALD Family Support Trust
30–32 Morley House
320 Regent Street
London W1R 5AB
Tel: 020 7631 3336
E-mail: info@aldfst.org.uk
www.aldfst.org.uk

Logophobia (fear of speaking) see Speech disorder

Low vision see Visual impairment

Lymphoma

Lymphoma is a cancer of the immune system that produces swellings of the lymph glands and can invade the bone marrow. The majority of children can now be treated successfully, although both the disease and its treatment carry heavy emotional and psychological burdens for the child and family. Treatments can produce immune deficiency, hair loss and later learning problems.

Children with lymphoma can be educated in mainstream and special schools. The extent to which lymphoma affects education depends on the medical interventions required. School-based *Interdisciplinary working* might be necessary for some children, while community medical services will manage others. Effective links with parents and good pastoral arrangements will provide support for these children through periods of treatment. Lymphoma may mean some children experience long and frequent periods of illness together with complex courses of treatment. Frequent absence from school for time-consuming treatments can lead to staff having low expectations of children's achievements and school friendships will be disrupted. It is important to explore all possible ways of supporting children who are regularly absent and to provide a range of ways to help them catch up with work; this becomes very important where children are mid-syllabus for externally accredited examinations. It is likely that education can be continued by hospital schools and attendant outreach teams.

Useful links
Lymphoma Association
PO Box 386
Aylesbury HP20 2GA
Tel: 0808 808 5555 and 01296 619400
www.lymphoma.org.uk

M

Macrocephaly

Macrocephaly means large head. This often runs in families and the child is entirely normal. In other cases the head is enlarged because of abnormalities of the brain and central nervous system within the skull – for example children with *Hydrocephalus* may have this condition.

Some children with macrocephaly can be educated in mainstream schools requiring additional help in the classroom because of their specific learning disabilities; others will need to attend special schools. School-based *Interdisciplinary working* involving therapists might be necessary for some children, while community medical services will manage others. Effective links with parents and good pastoral arrangements will provide support for these children.

The educational arrangements for children with this condition will vary widely between individuals. Children who have a significantly larger head than their peers will need support and care (see *Disfigurement and difference*). These children can have delayed development and language problems such as echoing of words and phrases (*Echolalia*), verbal processing difficulties, word finding problems, stammering, and difficulty controlling the muscles involved in vocal production (see *Speech and language problems*). They can experience clumsiness, an unsteady gait and poor coordination (see *Physical disability*). They can have difficulties with short-term memory, learning abstract ideas, practical reasoning, and numeracy and writing ability.

Some children can be aggressive and have challenging behaviours likely to arise from communication frustration, interaction difficulties, poor peer relationships and emotional immaturity. It is sensible to organise support mechanisms and management strategies to address known triggers or patterns that lead to conflict. Overall children with macrocephaly have a condition that may require some modification to elements of the curriculum.

Useful links
Child Growth Foundation
2 Mightfield Avenue
Chiswick
London W4 1PW
Tel: 020 8995 0257

Macular dystrophy *see* Retinitis pigmentosa

Marble-bone disease *see* Osteopetrosis

Marfan's syndrome

Marfan's syndrome is an inherited condition that affects growth in childhood, often making the child excessively tall. It is caused by a genetic problem in the formation of the connective tissues of the body. Affected children can have visual problems, heart problems and musculoskeletal difficulties.

Children with Marfan's syndrome can be educated in mainstream and special schools. The extent to which this condition affects schooling depends on the medical interventions required. Most will have their condition managed by community medical services. Effective links with parents and good pastoral arrangements will provide support for these children if necessary. Children with Marfan's syndrome will need access to the same curriculum as their peers (see *Visual impairment* and *Physical disability*). It is not unusual for children with Marfan's syndrome to be easily distracted, restless and at times impulsive (see *Attention deficit hyperactivity disorder*). The advice of medical professionals might be needed to ensure that exercises, activities and games in PE are appropriate.

Useful links

Hypermobility Syndrome Association
15 Oakdene
Alton GU34 2AJ
E-mail: info@hypermobility.org
www.hypermobility.org

Marfan Association UK
Rochester House
5 Aldershot Road
Fleet GU13 9NG
Tel: 01252 810472
E-mail: marfan@tinyonline.co.uk
www.marfan.org.uk

Maroteaux–Lamy syndrome *see* Mucopolysaccharidosis

ME (Myalgic encephalomyelitis) *see* Chronic fatigue syndrome

MELAS *see* Mitochondrial cytopathies

Meningitis

Meningitis is an inflammation of the outer lining of the brain and spinal cord. It can occur in clusters in schools and, where this is the case, antibiotic treatments to prevent infection (antibiotic prophylaxis) could be suggested. The illness can be treated successfully in most cases, particularly if recognised early. Children with meningitis may require intensive care in hospital and the infection is potentially life-threatening. The inflammation of the meninges can potentially damage the brain and some children will have a range of disabilities following the illness. Some children can have hearing difficulties, while others might have more widespread problems. Some forms of meningitis are also accompanied by blood poisoning (septicaemia), which can lead to kidney failure and amputations. When the brain itself is infected and becomes inflamed the child is said to have encephalitis.

Children who have had meningitis can be educated in mainstream and special schools. Children can experience a range of mild to severe consequences with a range of educational implications (see *Cerebral palsy, Epilepsy, Hydrocephalus, Visual impairment, Head injury* and *Hearing impairment*). School-based *Interdisciplinary working* involving therapists and specialist workers might be necessary for some children, while others will have their condition managed by community medical services. Effective links with parents and good pastoral arrangements will provide support for these children.

Children who have had meningitis will

need access to the same curriculum as their peers. Some children will spend long periods in wheelchairs, therefore access to classrooms and other school buildings needs to be good. Detailed work requiring fine motor skills should be adapted – some children cannot hold pencils easily and may need specialised keyboard access. The advice of medical professionals might be needed to ensure that exercises, activities and games in PE are appropriate.

Useful links
Meningitis Research Foundation
Unit 9 Thornbury Office Park
Midland Way
Thornbury
Bristol BS35 2BS
Tel: 080 8800 3344
E-mail: info@meningitis.org.uk
www.meningitis.org

National Meningitis Trust
Fern House
Bath Road
Stroud GL5 3TJ
Tel: 0845 6000 800
E-mail: support@meningitis-trust.org.uk
Website www.meningitis-trust.org.uk

MERRF syndrome *see* Mitochondrial cytopathies

Mesenteric adenitis *see* Appendicitis

Metachromatic leukodystrophy *see* Leukodystrophies

Microcephaly

Microcephaly means small head. It sometimes runs in families. Often the child is entirely normal, but in other cases the reason for the small head is that the brain underneath is not developing and growing properly. This can cause the skull bones to fuse together prematurely, a condition known as synostosis. In these cases the child can have a range of neurological, movement and developmental problems.

Children with microcephaly can be educated in mainstream and special schools. The educational arrangements for children with this condition will vary widely between individuals. School-based *Interdisciplinary working* involving therapists might be necessary for some children to provide strategies and approaches designed to give access to the curriculum, while others will have their condition managed based on community medical services. Effective links with parents and good pastoral arrangements will provide support for these children. A modified curriculum will be required for most children; for others a highly differentiated curriculum with high levels of individual attention will be required. Most difficulties are with mobility, fine motor activity, coordination and attention span. An individual educational programme should be designed to include movement skills, expressive and receptive communication. It will also need to promote the skills of self-help, independence, as well as social and daily living skills (see *Physical disability*).
Useful links

Child Growth Foundation
2 Mightfield Avenue
Chiswick
London W4 1PW
Tel: 020 8995 0257

Microphthalmia

Microphthalmia is the name given when the eye is abnormally small. It usually occurs as a congenital problem and there is reduced or absent vision in the affected eye. Other defects of the face or central nervous system can also occur, meaning that these children have other difficulties in addition to the obvious visual problems.

Children with microphthalmia can be educated in mainstream and special schools. School-based *Interdisciplinary working* might be necessary for some children, while community medical services will manage others. For further advice see *Visual impairment* and *Blindness*. Some children's appearance can be adversely affected (see *Disfigurement and difference*). Generally children with microphthalmia need a highly specialised curriculum.

Useful links
Hands and Eyes
A USA specialist teacher maintains this useful online newsletter for teachers and caregivers of visually impaired students and their friends. It includes art, cooking and manipulative activities that visually impaired students can do individually or in small groups. It is for teachers and support staff in need of ideas for classroom activities and is particularly useful for pupils with multiple impairments such as developmental disability and motor impairment.

www.home.earthlink.net/~vharris/

The Micro & Anophthalmic Childrens Society
1 Skyrmans
Frinton On Sea CO13 0RN
Tel/Fax: 01255 677511
E-mail: macs.uk@btInternet.com
http://webspace.dial.pipex.com/rbinfo/

RNIB Education Information Services
224 Great Portland Street
London W1N 6AA
Tel: 020 7388 1266
E-mail: webmaster@rnib.org.uk
www.rnib.org.uk
RNIB's curriculum information service offers information and advice to all professionals supporting a visually impaired child in mainstream or special schools.
www.rnib.org.uk/curriculum/
RNIB's accessing technology pages provide information about applications of technology in employment, at study and in leisure.
www.rnib.org.uk/technology/

V.I. Guide
This site contains information on many topics relating to parenting and teaching a child with visual impairments.
www.viguide.com/

Microstomia

Microstomia is usually a congenital defect in which the child has a mouth that is unusually small. On rare occasions children can have small mouths as a result of an accident. Children can have hard and tight skin or scar tissue around the face and mouth area. Tongue movement and therefore speech can be severely impaired. Reparative surgery takes some time and might involve frequent hospital visits (see the advice in *Disfigurement and difference*).

School-based *Interdisciplinary working* including the input of a speech and language therapist may be necessary for some children, while community medical services will manage others. Effective links with parents and good pastoral arrangements will provide support for these children. The advice in *Speech and language problems* will apply. Frequent absence from school for time-consuming treatments can lead to staff having low expectations of children's achievements and school friendships will be disrupted. It is important to explore all possible ways of supporting children who are regularly absent and to provide a range of ways to help them catch up with work; this becomes very important where children are mid-syllabus for externally accredited examinations. It is unlikely that the curriculum should be modified for children because they have microstomia.

Microtia *see* Treacher Collins syndrome

Migraine

Migraine occurs in children and can produce all the symptoms seen in adults. Children can sometimes feel the pain in their abdomen rather than as a headache. This is called *Abdominal migraine* (see entry). Children can also get visual disturbance, nausea, vomiting and a dislike of bright lights or loud noises

with the migraine.

Children who have migraines will show a wide range of reactions that can be easily misinterpreted. It is a complicated condition varying widely between individuals. The triggers or combinations of factors involved in attacks are individual, and symptoms will vary not only from child to child but from attack to attack in the same child. Severely affected children will be unable to work as well as their peers and need to have special arrangements for opportunities to learn outside the conventional school day. Some children will need access to a quiet haven and the possibility of a short sleep. Maintaining close liaison with parents is very helpful as they may have some idea of precipitants and effective treatments.

Where the likely causes of migraine are known, then avoidance strategies can be used. Migraines can follow change of sleep routine, stress, fatigue, exertion, excitement, dietary and hormone changes, and missing meals. It is helpful to work closely with a child and encourage them to learn about their condition and those things that they can do to manage it. The curriculum should not need to be modified for children because they have migraines; however, some children will be absent from school while recovering.

Useful links
The Migraine Trust
45 Great Ormond Street
London WC1N 3HZ
Tel: 020 7831 4818
www.migrainetrust.org

Minimal brain dysfunction

This general term can be used where the patterns of development, learning, thought and action of children are those found in an organic disorder, but one is not evident. Children are more often described as having *Dyspraxia*, *Attention deficit disorder* and *Attention deficit hyperactivity disorder*, hyperkinetic syndrome, impulsivity, and signs of a number of learning and language disabilities such as *Dyslexia* and *Dyscalculia*. For further information see *Specific learning difficulties*.

Mitochondrial cytopathies

Mitochondrial cytopathies are a group of conditions where the underlying problem occurs in the mitochondria of the child's cells. These parts of the cell provide energy for normal cellular functioning. As they are present in virtually all the cells of the body, any or many body systems can be involved. Leber's optic atrophy, Kearns–Sayre syndrome, Leigh's disease, MERRF syndrome and MELAS are all examples of this type of disorder. Many give rise to visual problems, muscle weakness, epilepsy and learning difficulties.

Some children with mitochondrial cytopathies have their educational needs met in mainstream schools, while others will need very special care and the highly differentiated education usually found in a special school. School-based *Interdisciplinary working* involving therapists might be necessary for some children, while others will have their condition managed based on community medical services. Effective links with parents and good pastoral arrangements will provide support for these children.

Children with mitochondrial cytopathies will need access to the same curriculum as their peers. The curriculum might need highly specialised input from experienced and trained specialist teachers (see *Physical disability*, *Visual impairment*, *Hearing impairment*). Overall, children with mitochondrial cytopathies have a condition that will significantly affect their education.

Useful links
Climb
The Quadrangle
Crewe Hall
Weston Road
Crewe CW2 6UR
Tel: 0870 770 0326
E-mail: info@climb.org.uk
www.climb.org.uk

Mixed hearing loss

Mixed hearing loss causes difficulty as the conductive component can fluctuate and the child's behaviour can vary from day to day. Since mixed losses combine the characteristics of conductive and sensorineural loss, the extent of each component will determine the degree of loss.

Children with mixed hearing loss can be educated in mainstream and special schools. School-based *Interdisciplinary working* involving specialist teachers, audiologists and audio technicians might be necessary for some children, while community medical services will manage others. Effective links with parents and good pastoral arrangements will provide support for these children. The advice found under *Hearing impairment* will apply.

Moebius syndrome

Moebius syndrome causes weakness of some of the muscles of the head, neck and face. This can affect feeding, swallowing, speech and vision. Children have an expressionless face from nerve weakness and can have developmental or learning difficulties. The arms and hands can also be abnormal.

Children with Moebius syndrome have difficulties communicating through facial expression. Because they are unable to smile or frown it can be difficult for staff to know whether the child is comfortable and therefore receptive to teaching and learning. School-based *Interdisciplinary working* will be necessary including the advice of specialist teachers and speech and language therapists in devising a means for children to communicate their current state or well-being. It is important to have an effective means of communicating with parents who will have developed tried and tested ways of communicating with their child. Good pastoral arrangements should be in place to support and to ensure that peers are aware of how the child communicates (see *Disfigurement and difference*). Class teams should develop recording and reporting strategies in order to monitor how effectively the child manages across the school day.

Some children can have a number of associated difficulties including sensitive vision (due to inability in some to blink), upper body fatigue, difficulties with eating and with producing clear speech. PE activities might need to be modified or limited. Children with Moebius syndrome will need careful support in all areas of the curriculum.

Monoplegia *see* Cerebral palsy

Morquio disease *see* Mucopolysaccharidosis

Motor dyspraxia *see* Dyspraxia

Mucopolysaccharidosis

Mucopolysaccharidosis is the name given to a group of rare congenital conditions where vital chemicals (enzymes) that help the body's cells maintain themselves are missing. The result is a build-up of unwanted cellular waste products that over time can cause damage and increasing disability. There are six main conditions in this group: Hurler disease, Hunter disease, Sanfillipo syndrome, Morquio disease, Maroteaux–Lamy syndrome and Sly syndrome. They cause growth problems, coarsening of the child's features, short stature, *Scoliosis* (a progressive bend in the back), visual problems, enlargement of the liver and spleen and (in some conditions) progressive learning difficulties and cognitive impairment.

Children with mucopolysaccharidosis can initially have their educational needs met in mainstream schools, but inevitably the progress of the condition will mean that they need very special care and a highly differentiated education. The educational programme will need to include the maintenance of skills and providing the same curriculum entitlements of all children. As time goes by school-based *Interdisciplinary working* involving therapists will become necessary (see *Physical disability*, *Visual impairment*). The school will need to have an excellent pastoral policy and practice, giving the children and their family high levels of support and counselling. Overall children with mucopolysaccharidosis have a condition that will significantly affect their education.

Useful links
The Society for Mucopolysaccharide Diseases
46 Woodside Road
Amersham HP6 6AJ
Tel: 01494 434156
E-mail: mps@mpssociety.co.uk
www.mpssociety.co.uk

Multisensory impairment *see* Deafblind

Mutism (a child's choice or inability to speak due to psychological factors) *see* Elective mutism

Myalgic encephalomyelitis (ME) *see* Chronic fatigue syndrome

Myocarditis *see* Cardiomyopathies

Myopia *see* Refractive error

N

Naevus flammeus *see* Port-wine stain

Nephrotic syndrome

Nephrotic syndrome is a condition that causes the kidneys to lose excessive amounts of protein into the urine. The loss of protein can cause extensive swelling and the child can become very unwell during an attack. As some of the proteins lost by the kidneys are those involved in providing the child with normal immunity, the child is at increased risk of developing severe infections. Treatment is usually with steroids, although other drugs are also used. The condition can recur. The swelling that accompanies the attack can be quite disfiguring for the child (see *Disfigurement and difference*).

Children with nephrotic syndrome can be educated in mainstream and special schools. Most children will have their condition managed by community medical services. Effective links with parents and good pastoral arrangements will provide the child with support. Frequent absence from school and time-consuming treatments can lead to staff having low expectations of the child. It is important to explore all possible ways of supporting children who are regularly absent and to provide a range of ways to help them catch up with work; this becomes very important where children are mid-syllabus for externally accredited examinations. It is unlikely that the curriculum should be modified for children because they have a nephrotic syndrome; however, some children are absent from school while receiving treatment.

Useful links
National Kidney Federation
6 Stanley Street
Worksop
Notts S81 7HX
Tel: 0845 601 0209
E-mail: helpline@kidney.org.uk
www.kidney.org.uk

Nephronline
E-mail: info@nephronline.org
www.nephronline.org/

Nerve deafness *see* Sensorineural hearing loss

Neurofibromatosis

Neurofibromatosis causes patches of pigment (café au lait patches) to appear on a child's skin. Learning difficulties can also be present and there is a risk of high blood pressure and *Scoliosis*. Memory can be affected and the child can have problems with inattentiveness and impulsivity. Abnormal growths on nerve tissue are the cause of some of the problems. Rarely the nerve from the eyes to the brain can be affected. Older children and adults can also be affected similarly, sometimes giving rise to growths that affect the nerves from the ears to the brain.

Children with neurofibromatosis can be educated in mainstream and special schools. Good pastoral support arrangements and school-based *Interdisciplinary working* will be important. Some children can look very different (see *Disfigurement and difference*) and can also have visual impairment and hearing loss leading to communication difficulties.

Many children manage to access the mainstream curriculum with support while others require more specialist provision. Children might need support in all formal academic areas such as reading, writing, listening and mathematics. Some children will have difficulty with visualising objects in relation to each other, with memory, organisation, visual processing and motor coordination. These problems can lead to poor performance in mathematics, geometry, and tasks requiring manual dexterity or sense of direction. Some children have poor self-esteem leading to difficult and antisocial behaviours. Overall, children with neurofibromatosis have a condition that will to some extent affect their education.

Useful links
The Neurofibromatosis Association
82 London Road
Kingston upon Thames KT2 6PX
Tel: 020 8547 1636
E-mail: nfa@zetnet.co.uk
www.nfa.zetnet.co.uk

Neuropathic bladder

Neuropathic bladder is the condition where the nerves that control and coordinate the evacuation of the bladder are faulty and result in uncoordinated emptying: failure of the bladder to empty when full or sudden emptying of the bladder without warning. All these problems can occur without the child having the feeling that the bladder is full and they might be unaware that they are passing urine until wetness is seen or felt. Treatment can be with drugs and sometimes with catheterisation or even surgery. Children with *Spina bifida* often have this condition.

For the child with wetting due to neuropathic bladder, these problems can lead to blame at home, bullying at school (if the child smells of stale urine) and thereby to low self-esteem. Where staff are aware that children are wetting during the school day, then special care arrangements might be needed in order to manage the situation effectively without drawing the unnecessary attention of peers. As wetting is very obvious, staff will need to develop ways of monitoring children to prevent inappropriate comments and/or bullying.

Children who wet themselves have their educational needs met in mainstream and special schools. School-based *Interdisciplinary working* might be necessary for some children; others will have their condition managed by community medical services. Effective links with parents and good pastoral arrangements will provide the child with support. It is unlikely that the curriculum should be modified for children because they are wetting during the school day. However, it is likely that some measures may be needed to prevent adverse reactions that can lead to low self-esteem and poor school work.

Useful links
Bedwetting.co.uk
4 Harforde Court
John Tate Road
Hertford SG13 7NW
Tel: 01992 526300
E-mail: info@bedwetting.co.uk
www.bedwetting.co.uk/nhsnews.htm

The Enuresis Resource & Information
Centre
34 Old School House
Britannia Road
Kingswood
Bristol BS15 8DB
Tel: 0117 960 3060
E-mail: info@eric.org.uk
www.enuresis.org.uk

Nocturnal enuresis

Nocturnal enuresis occurs in many school-aged children and is the involuntary passing of urine overnight while the child sleeps. Most children with nocturnal enuresis are perfectly healthy and the condition merely reflects the later development of this aspect of continence. Virtually all children will grow out of this. 'Treatment' can be undertaken with behavioural approaches, avoiding drinks that contain caffeine, use of alarms that go off when the child passes urine and medication to reduce the amount of urine that the kidneys make overnight.

For the child, bedwetting can lead to blame at home, bullying at school (if the child comes to school smelling of stale urine) and thereby to low self-esteem. If evidence of wetting is very obvious, staff will need to develop ways of monitoring children to prevent inappropriate comments and/or bullying.

Children who wet at night have their educational needs met in mainstream and special schools. School-based *Interdisciplinary working* might help some children, although most children will have their condition managed by community medical services. Effective links with parents and good pastoral arrangements will provide the child with support. The curriculum will not need to be modified for children because they are wet at night.

Useful links
Bedwetting.co.uk
4 Harforde Court
John Tate Road
Hertford SG13 7NW
Tel: 01992 526300
E-mail: info@bedwetting.co.uk
www.bedwetting.co.uk/nhsnews.htm

The Enuresis Resource & Information
Centre
34 Old School House
Britannia Road
Kingswood
Bristol BS15 8DB
Tel: 0117 960 3060
E-mail: info@eric.org.uk
www.enuresis.org.uk

Noonan syndrome

Noonan syndrome is a condition where children are short, may have heart defects, hearing and visual difficulties, fertility problems, clotting problems, and also learning and speech difficulties.

Children with Noonan syndrome can be educated in all schools, dependant on the degree to which they are affected. School-based *Interdisciplinary working* will be necessary including the advice of specialist teachers, speech and language therapists and possibly an educational psychologist.

Some children have difficulties with speech and will need to have regular opportunities to work on exercises designed by speech and language therapists. Other children will have better nonverbal than verbal skills. Some children will have difficulty visualising objects in relation to each other, with visual memory and with visual–motor coordination. This problem can lead to poor performance in mathematics, geometry, and tasks requiring manual dexterity or sense of direction. A small number of children have hearing loss (see *Hearing impairment*). Generally children with Noonan syndrome have a condition that will require some modification to their educational provision.

Nystagmus

Nystagmus is a problem affecting the eyes that causes them to oscillate. This can affect vision or can in turn be caused by defects in the development of the eyesight. Some cases are noticed soon after birth (known as congenital nystagmus), while others develop nystagmus after a few months and it might be just part of the child's more extensive visual problems (see *Albinism* and *Achromatopsia*).

Children with nystagmus can be educated in mainstream and special schools. The extent to which this condition affects schooling depends on how severely eye movement is affected. School-based *Interdisciplinary working* involving a specialist teacher for visual impairment might be necessary for some children, while others will have their condition managed by community medical services. Effective links with parents and good pastoral arrangements will provide support for these children.

Problems with vision can affect development of movement, coordination and speech. For further information see *Visual impairment*.

Useful links
Nystagmus Network
76 Midland Road
Cotteridge
Birmingham B30 2EY
Tel: 01392 272573
E-mail: NystagmusN@aol.com

O

Oesophagitis *see* Abdominal pain

Oligoarthritis

Oligoarthritis is the term for when arthritis has been present in four or fewer joints during the first six months after the onset of symptoms. It is the commonest form of arthritis in young children with girls more commonly affected than boys. It does not usually affect the same joint on both sides of the body. Early indications of oligoarthritis could be reluctance in using a joint or part of the body or a limp; some children do not indicate any discomfort or pain. Oligoarthritis is associated with an eye condition called uveitis or chronic iridocyclitis. If undetected and untreated, this condition can cause severe eye damage; it is therefore essential that the child's eyes are checked regularly by an ophthalmologist even after the oligoarthritis has disappeared. Over time most children with oligoarthritis improve and recurrences are unusual. If some joints remain swollen, then the condition is known as persistent oligoarthritis.

Children with oligoarthritis will have their educational needs met in mainstream and special schools. The extent to which this condition affects schooling will be dependant on how the condition restricts the child's mobility. School-based *Interdisciplinary working* may be necessary for some children; others will have their condition managed by community medical services. Effective links with parents and good pastoral arrangements will provide children with support.

Children with oligoarthritis will need access to the same curriculum as their peers. The advice of medical professionals might be needed to ensure that exercises, activities and games in PE are appropriate. Overall, children with oligoarthritis have a condition that is unlikely to interfere with their education.

Useful links
Arthritis Care Youth Service
The Source, 18 Stephenson Way
London NW1 2HD
Tel 0808 808 2000
E-mail: thesource@arthritiscare.org.uk
www.arthritiscare.org.uk

Children's Chronic Arthritis Association
Ground Floor Office
Amber Gate, City Walls Road
Worcester WR1 2AH
Tel: 01905 745595

Oppositional defiant disorder *see* Conduct disorder or disruptive behaviour disorder

Optic atrophy/Optic nerve hypoplasia

In these conditions, the nerve that takes the impulses generated by the retina is damaged or underdeveloped. Optic atrophy can result from raised intracranial pressure and can lead to visual loss. Children with optic nerve hypoplasia can have visual difficulties relating to the way the brain interprets visual signals from the eyes (see *Cortical blindness*). Children with optic atrophy will experience varying degrees of impairment from normal to severely impaired. For further advice see *Visual impairment*. Children with optic atrophy can be educated in mainstream and special schools. School-based *Interdisciplinary working* will be necessary including the advice of a specialist teacher for visual impairment in the planning of an effective educational programme. Enhancing visual function may require high levels of illumination and enlarged print with high contrast; magnification can be useful in some cases. For some children distinguishing between colours can be a problem – this will clearly have implications across the curriculum. The day-to-day classroom performance of a student with optic atrophy may vary for no apparent reason; the classroom teacher will therefore need to be prepared to make necessary adaptations to short-term plans.

Useful links
Hands and Eyes
A USA specialist teacher maintains this useful online newsletter for teachers and caregivers of visually impaired students and their friends. It includes art, cooking and manipulative activities that visually impaired students can do individually or in small groups. It is for teachers and support staff in need of ideas for classroom activities and is particularly useful for pupils with multiple impairments such as developmental disability and motor impairment.
www.home.earthlink.net/~vharris/

RNIB Education Information Services
224 Great Portland Street
London W1N 6AA
Tel: 020 7388 1266
E-mail: webmaster@rnib.org.uk
www.rnib.org.uk
RNIB's curriculum information service offers infor-

mation and advice to all professionals supporting a visually impaired child in mainstream or special schools.
www.rnib.org.uk/curriculum/
RNIB's accessing technology pages provide information about applications of technology in employment, at study and in leisure.
www.rnib.org.uk/technology/

V.I. Guide
This site contains information on many topics relating to parenting and teaching a child with visual impairments.
www.viguide.com/

Osteogenesis imperfecta see Brittle bone disease

Osteomyelitis

Osteomyelitis and septic arthritis are infections of the bones and joints respectively. They can cause fever, pain and deformity. Both conditions need treatment with antibiotics and might require surgery; treatment is sometimes lengthy, leading to time off school. Mobility, self-care and manipulative abilities can be adversely affected.

Children with arthritis can be educated in mainstream and special schools. The extent to which this condition affects schooling depends on severity and the medical interventions required. For some children pain management is important; others experience long periods of restricted mobility and will need exercises designed by a physiotherapist. School-based *Interdisciplinary working* involving a physiotherapist and an occupational therapist might be necessary for some children, while others will have their condition managed by medical services. Effective links with parents and good pastoral arrangements will provide the child with support.

Children with septic arthritis will need access to the same curriculum as their peers. Children in the primary phase may need special attention; they might not tell staff when there is discomfort or a problem, because they are engrossed in a particular activity or because they might prefer to avoid treatment. Some children will temporarily need wheelchairs, therefore access to classrooms and the building needs to be good (see *Physical disability*). The advice of medical professionals might be needed to ensure that exercises, activities and games in PE are appropriate. Overall, children with septic arthritis have a condition that can sometimes interfere with their education.

Useful links
Arthritis Research Campaign
Copeman House
St Mary's Court
St Mary's Gate
Chesterfield
Derbyshire S41 7TD
E-mail: info@arc.org.uk
www.arc.org.uk

Osteopetrosis

Osteopetrosis occurs when the bones are abnormally thick. The thickening causes the bone marrow (which manufactures red and white blood cells) to become obliterated. The child has anaemia or immunity problems. They can also have low calcium levels. In some cases of early-onset disease, the thickening skull bones damage the nerve from the eye causing blindness. The abnormal bone can fracture.

Treatment is aimed at monitoring the vision and ensuring anaemia is treated adequately. The condition can be life-threatening, particularly when it affects very young children.

Children with osteopetrosis can be educated in mainstream and special schools. The extent to which this condition affects schooling depends on the way the condition progresses. Some children will experience a number of long periods of restricted mobility and will need exercises designed by a physiotherapist. School-based *Interdisciplinary working* involving a physiotherapist and an occupational therapist might be necessary for some children, while others will have their condition managed by community medical services. Effective links with parents and good pastoral arrangements will provide the child with support.

Some children can be severely affected and need very special care and education (see *Visual impairment* and *Physical disability*). The educational programme will include maintenance of skills and providing the same entitlements of all children. As time goes by the curriculum will increasingly need to be highly differentiated.

Useful links
Osteopetrosis Support Trust – OST
10 Cumberland Avenue
Fixby
Huddersfield HD2 2JJ
Tel: 01484 545974
E-mail: magken@mwright86.fsnet.co.uk
www.ost.org.uk

Osteoporosis

Osteoporosis is the condition where the bones lack calcium and therefore become weak. The child is liable to suffer fractures, particularly of the spinal column. Children taking large doses, or long-term courses of steroids are at risk of developing the condition. Children with *Osteogenesis imperfecta* have osteoporotic bones. Pain and immobility are the main consequences of the condition.

Children with osteoporosis can be educated in mainstream and special schools. The extent to which this condition affects schooling depends on medical advice and the outcomes of risk assessments. School-based *Interdisciplinary working* involving a physiotherapist and an occupational therapist might be necessary for some children, while others will have their condition managed by community medical services. Effective links with parents and good pastoral arrangements will provide the child with support.

Children with osteoporosis will need access to the same curriculum as their peers. The advice of medical professionals might be needed to ensure that exercises, activities and games in PE are appropriate. Running, aerobics, tennis, weight-training and skipping are usually considered beneficial as they will help stimulate bone strength.

Useful links
Osteoporosis Society
PO Box 10
Radstock
Bath BA3 3YB
Tel: 01761 472721
Helpline: 01761 471771

Fax: 01761 471104
E-mail: info@nos.org.uk
www.nos.org.uk

Osteosarcoma

Osteosarcoma is a cancer of the bones. It can cause pain, swelling or a fracture. Affected children require chemotherapy and may also need surgery. Children with osteosarcoma can be educated in mainstream and special schools. The extent to which this condition affects schooling depends on its severity and the medical interventions required. For some children pain management is important; others experience long periods of restricted mobility and will need exercises designed by a physiotherapist. School-based *Interdisciplinary working* involving a physiotherapist and an occupational therapist might be necessary for some children, while community medical services will manage others. Effective links with parents and good pastoral arrangements will provide the child with support.

Children with osteosarcoma will need access to the same curriculum as their peers. Some children will temporarily need wheelchairs, therefore access to classrooms and the building needs to be good (see *Physical disability*). The advice of medical professionals might be needed to ensure that exercises, activities and games in PE are appropriate. Overall, children with osteosarcoma have a temporary condition that can interfere with their education.

Useful links
Cancer Research UK

National Office
61 Lincoln's Inn Fields
London WC2A 3PX
Tel: 020 7242 0200
www.cancerhelp.org.uk

Otitis externa

Otitis externa is inflammation of the outside parts of the ears. It is very painful for the child and is treated with antibiotics and sometimes steroids. It is usually only a temporary problem. Children with otitis externa can be educated in mainstream and special schools. Effective links with parents and good pastoral arrangements will provide children with care and support. Some children are temporarily unable to participate in some physical activities, such as swimming. It is unlikely that the curriculum should be modified for children because they have otitis externa.

Otitis media

Otitis media is the inflammation of the middle ear (the part of the ear immediately behind the eardrum). It is a very common childhood illness that occurs in younger children producing a fever and pain in the ear (acute otitis media). It is often treated with antibiotics. It can result in the eardrum bursting and usually resolves without any problems. In some children the perforation does not heal (chronic otitis media) and this leads to longer-lasting problems with discharges from the ears and hearing loss. In serous otitis media or glue ear, the middle ear becomes painlessly congested with secretions that prevent the eardrum from vibrating freely. This causes a fluctuating hearing loss. As it often occurs in younger children who are developing language, it is often looked for as a cause of language delay. Many cases improve spontaneously over time, but many children are treated by the insertion of *Grommets*. For children whose hearing is compromised by these conditions, communication, access to aural work and development of language are all potentially affected.

Children with otitis media can be educated in mainstream and special schools. School-based *Interdisciplinary working* involving specialist teachers, audiologists and audio technicians might be necessary for some children, while community medical services will manage others. Effective links with parents and good pastoral arrangements will provide support for these children. The advice found under *Hearing impairment* will apply.

Most children will let parents or significant adults know if their ear hurts, but some will not. Observation through the school day will provide information that could indicate ear infection. Children may demonstrate discomfort in a variety of ways by crying and holding their head, tugging or pulling at ears, not keeping their balance, not responding to quiet sounds, etc. In some children fluid can be seen draining out of the ears. Staff need to be vigilant and ensure common sense approaches, such as not placing children where there is noisy equipment or deliberately sitting children near the teacher. It is also helpful to systematically check for understanding and learning, making sure children see those who are speaking and ensuring those that speak do so clearly. Should a child's speech become unclear staff should contact parents recommending a visit to their General Practitioner for possible referral to an audiologist to check hearing or to a speech and language therapist.

Useful links
deafPLUS
Prospect Hall
12 College Walk
Selly Oak
Birmingham B29 6LE
Tel: 0171 415 2080
E-mail: info@deafPLUS.org
www.deafplus.org

The National Deaf Children's Society
15 Dufferin Street
London EC1Y 8UR
Tel: 020 7490 8656
Helpline: 020 7250 0123
E-mail: fundraising@ndcs.org.uk
www.ncds.org.uk
RNID

19–23 Featherstone Street
London EC1Y 8SL
Tel: 0808 808 123
E-mail: informationline@rnid.org.uk
www.rnid.org.uk

Otosclerosis

Otosclerosis is a thickening of the bones of the middle ear that conduct vibrations from the eardrum to the inner ear. It leads to a *Conductive hearing loss*. Some children find a *Hearing aid* helpful. Dependant on the extent of hearing loss, the advice found under *Hearing impairment* will apply. Children with otosclerosis can be educated in mainstream and special schools. School-based *Interdisciplinary working* involving specialist teachers, audiologists and audio technicians might be necessary for some children, while community medical services will manage others. Effective links with parents and good pastoral arrangements will provide support for these children.

P

Patent ductus arteriosus (PDA)

PDA occurs when the connection between the two main arteries that leave the heart remains open after the birth of the child. This results in extra blood flowing through the lungs. Small PDAs rarely cause symptoms during childhood, although larger defects can cause breathlessness and, in young children, growth difficulties. The flow of blood through the hole can increase the risk of infections in the heart (endocarditis). The hole rarely closes off on its own, but can be closed off by an operation, or through a flexible tube (catheter). This condition can coexist with other heart defects.

For the child at school, the main impact of a large defect will be on their ability to take part in strenuous physical exercise (see *Congenital heart diseases*).

Pauciarticular arthritis *see* Oligoarthritis

Pediculosis *see* Head lice

Pendred syndrome

Pendred syndrome causes thyroid gland problems (see *Hypothyroidism*) and *Hearing impairment*. The hearing loss can be severe and permanent.

Children with Pendred syndrome can be educated in mainstream and special schools. School-based *Interdisciplinary working* including the advice of specialist teachers, therapists and possibly an educational psychologist might be necessary for some children, while community medical services will manage others. Careful liaison with parents and carers and effective pastoral support arrangements should be in place to support the child.

For those children who experience hearing loss the advice found under *Hearing impairment* will apply. The impact of any hearing loss should be monitored and will need basic attention, such as:

- not placing the child where there is noisy equipment
- sitting the child near the teacher
- systematic checking for understanding and learning
- making sure the child sees those who are speaking and ensuring those that speak do so clearly.

Children with hearing loss may present classroom behaviour problems and appear to not pay attention.

Peroxisomal disorder *see* Zellweger syndrome

Persistent ductus arteriosus *see* Patent ductus arteriosus

Perthes disease

Perthes disease affects the hip joints and is caused by problems with the blood supply to the head of the thigh bone as it sits within the socket of the hip joint. This in turn causes destruction of the bony head and consequent pain and limitation of movement. Pain may be either felt in the hip or referred to the knees. It mostly occurs in boys aged between 2 and 10 years and can lead to prolonged immobility and in some cases wheelchair dependency whilst the disease is active. In most cases the joint recovers and full movement is restored.

In severely affected children, pain and restricted mobility may impact upon their ability to access the curriculum. Physiotherapy is often employed to ensure that function is maintained and then regained as quickly as possible. The advice and considerations about the school environment, curriculum and resources found under *Physical disability* will apply.

Useful links
Perthes Association
15 Recreation Road
Guildford
GU1 1HE
Tel: 01483 306637
E-mail: admin@perthes.org.uk
www.perthes.org.uk/

Phenylketonuria

Phenylketonuria is the congenital absence of an enzyme that uses and breaks down the amino acid phenylalanine in the diet. Phenylalanine is derived from protein and the condition leads to high levels of harmful chemicals produced by the incomplete breakdown of phenylalanine damaging the developing brain, nervous system and fertility. A special diet is needed, which becomes very difficult for children to follow once they are of school age.

Children with phenylketonuria can be educated in mainstream and special schools. School-based *Interdisciplinary working* will be necessary including the advice of medical advisers and dieticians. Staff in school should be scrupulous in ensuring the child's dietary needs are met. Good pastoral support arrangements should be in place to help the child. Careful liaison with parents and carers is important to ensure that dietary requirements are met across the whole day.

Some children will require a highly specialised educational environment with high staffing levels and a team skilled in the management of behaviour. The curriculum will need to be modified for some children because of problems with visualising objects in relation to each other owing to visual memory and visual–motor coordination difficulties. This problem can show up in poor performance in mathematics, geometry, and tasks requiring manual dexterity or sense of direction. Some children need an individual language and communication programme.

Useful links
National Society for Phenylketonuria (UK) Ltd
PO Box 26642
London N14 4ZF
Tel: 0845 603 9136
E-mail: nspku@ukonline.co.uk
http://web.ukonline.co.uk/nspku

Phimosis *see* Circumcision

Photophobia *see* Coloboma

Physical disability – generic advice only

The individual requirements to meet the special educational needs of children and young people with physical disabilities will usually be found in school records, the IEP, in the advice provided at assessment prior to a statement being issued or in the reports provided to an annual review of a statement.

Children with physical disabilities can be educated in mainstream and special schools. School-based *Interdisciplinary working* involving a physiotherapist and an occupational therapist might be necessary for some children, while community medical services will manage others. Effective links with parents and good pastoral arrangements will provide support for these children. Consideration and attention should be given to the environment, curriculum and resources; if these are not suitable, then adaptations should be considered.

Children with physical disabilities are often described by their disability, and not by their strengths or abilities. All children have characteristics or skills that are better than other abilities. School information about children should highlight strengths as well as provide factual information.

The extent to which a physical disability is a barrier to learning will vary considerably; different situations require specific solutions or adaptations. Prior to admission it is good practice to meet with the pupil and, if possible, their parents to help clarify individual needs. New pupils should be visited in their current school by staff from the new school well before the date of transfer. Much useful information can be gleaned from colleagues

with experience of working with the child. A specific transition plan should be designed, including relevant aims for each visit to their new school. Initially a child with a physical disability should be orientated within the new school to learn about ramps or lifts where available, and access to toilets and other areas. Once the child is in the school, it is important for him or her to form and maintain meaningful interpersonal relationships with their new classmates. Encourage the child to join in as many formal and informal classroom activities as possible. Try to ensure that appropriate arrangements are made so that the child can participate in activities that take place outside school. The child may need to have special arrangements made to take prescribed medication; the move to the child's independent management of their own medication might need monitoring and support.

Care and attention must be given to the child's ability to manage their bodily functions. Lack of bowel and bladder control is one of the barriers to social acceptance; accidents happen and incontinence equipment can fail. It is good practice to programme toilet breaks/checks towards the end of a session to avoid mid-session interruptions and to make sure that the child is included in breaks. It is helpful to set up systems to exchange information between home and school regularly to maintain shared understanding and consistency. Children usually enjoy involvement in this.

Ideally children should be taught in single-storey buildings located on accessible sites. Access across the school site needs to be good. An assessment or audit is useful – do not assume anything. If it is not possible to involve the new pupil, then seek the help of an adult with similar physical needs as this can provide good information quickly. Many arrangements and adaptations are compromises and often completed in haste. Do everything possible to plan ahead and give time for site works and building modifications. There should be large classrooms with wide doors and, for some children, additional workspaces for therapists and medical teams.

Specialised postural equipment could be needed together with equipment for lifting and transferring; this might need to be stored close to where needed. The involvement of an occupational therapist and a physiotherapist is important in advising on the right kind of seat or table and other postural equipment. Good seating and positioning aids learning. The child needs to be anchored with feet flat on the floor – sometimes it can be beneficial to have a seating wedge to transfer weight through the hips and to the feet. Tables are better at hip height and, for some children, an angle board can support an arm providing added stability to the upper torso. Anchoring legs and arms to help stabilise the pelvis and shoulders helps the child to sit still. The seat and table need to be positioned so that the child can easily see the teacher. In lessons the seated position can be convenient but not desirable for some pupils; standing for periods of time might be more beneficial but more problematic to organise.

Encourage as much physical activity as a physiotherapist recommends, as it is important for pupils with physical disabilities to remain as active as possible in order to keep in optimum condition. Access to a swimming or hydrotherapy pool with appropriate changing facilities can be of great benefit to those with the most complex physical disabilities.

Attention to communication is very important with some children using specialised communication aids (see *Alternative and augmentative communication*). Make sure that staff are familiar with equipment, such as adapted typewriters, pencil holders, book holders, page turners, word boards or special desks. Use handouts, tapes and other adapted media, to allow access and to enable children to keep pace with peers. Encourage the use of computers, typewriters and other aids to increase the capacity for written work and to overcome any difficulties of hand control. Support the pupil in completing work even if extra time is required. A task that has been accomplished will do much to raise self-esteem

Assist the student to develop organisational skills by keeping books and school materials within easy reach and by making lists and schedules of work, tests, special events, etc. Have high expectations of students including acceptable and appropriate behaviour. Students with disabilities need the same treatment and expectations as their classmates.

Some students require extensive medical support, which can be time-consuming, inconvenient and stressful. Frequent absence from school and time-consuming treatments can lead to low expectations. It is important to explore all possible ways of supporting children who are regularly absent and to provide a range of ways to help them catch up with work, particularly where children are mid-syllabus for externally accredited examinations.

Useful links
Contact a Family
209–211 City Road
London EC1V 1JN
Tel: 020 7608 8700
E-mail: info@cafamily.org.uk
www.cafamily.org.uk/index.html

DfES
Sanctuary Buildings
Great Smith Street
London SW1P 3BT
www.dfes.gov.uk/sen/index.cfm

NASEN
NASEN House
4/5 Amber Business Village
Amber Close
Amington
Tamworth B77 4RP
Tel: 01827 311500
E-mail: welcome@nasen.org.uk
www.nasen.org.uk/contact/

Pigeon toes *see* Intoeing

Pinworms *see* Worms

Pituitary disorders

Pituitary disorders can affect growth, puberty, metabolism, learning and behaviour. Any of these can be slowed down or speeded up depending on whether the pituitary gland is failing or overactive. The gland controls secretion of thyroid hormone (see *Hypothyroidism*, *Hyperthyroidism*), growth hormone (see *Growth hormone deficiency*), sex stimulating hormones, and hormones that stimulate the production of the body's own natural steroids (see *Cushing's syndrome*, including hypoadrenalism). Affected children can therefore experience difficulties with growth, puberty, behaviour and learning.

Children with pituitary disorders can be educated in mainstream and special schools; educational arrangements will vary widely between individuals. School-based *Interdisciplinary working* might be necessary for some children, while community medical services will manage others. Effective links with parents and good pastoral arrangements will provide support for these children.

Some children will spend time away from school in hospital. Good liaison between schools and hospital education services is important in order to support curriculum continuity. A school needs good systems of support and opportunities for children to catch up after periods of absence. Children needing frequent absence from school can lead to staff having low expectations of them and school friendships will be disrupted. It is important to explore all possible ways of supporting children who are absent for long periods and to provide a range of ways to help them catch up with work; this becomes very important where children are mid-syllabus for externally accredited examinations.

Useful links
The Pituitary Foundation
PO Box 1944
Bristol BS99 2UB
Tel/Fax: 0870 774 3355
E-mail: helpline@pituitary.org.uk
www.pituitary.org.uk

Plagiocephaly

Plagiocephaly is the term given to a misshapen head. It is relatively common (and most noticeable) in young babies, where the head looks squashed to one side. As the child grows and the hair lengthens, the deformity becomes less obvious. Severe plagiocephaly can be treated surgically. There are few educational implications.

Children with plagiocephaly can be educated in mainstream and special schools. Most children will have their condition managed by community medical services. Effective links with parents and good pastoral arrangements will be needed to provide the child with support. Some children can look very different and may need counselling (see *Disfigurement and difference*).

Children with plagiocephaly will need access to the same curriculum as their peers. It is unlikely that the curriculum should be modified for children because they have plagiocephaly.

Useful links
The Craniofacial Support Group
44 Helmsdale Road
Leamington Spa CV32 7DW
Tel: 01926 334629
www.craniofacial.org.uk/UKsupport.htm

Pneumonia

Pneumonia is an infection of the lung that affects the air sacs (alveoli). It is mainly due to bacteria and viruses. The illness causes shortness of breath, coughing and (some-times) wheezing. Bacterial infections are treated with antibiotics. Children can be left with a cough for some time (weeks and sometimes months) after the infection has been successfully treated.

This condition is usually managed by the family doctor and might include time in hospital or the interventions of community medical services. Effective links with parents and good pastoral arrangements might be needed. It is unlikely that the curriculum should be modified for children because they have pneumonia; however, some children will be absent from school while receiving treatment.

Polio

Polio is extremely rare in developed countries thanks to vaccination. However, children originating from third world countries may be affected. In its severest form it leads to severe weakness of the muscles used for breathing and necessitates long-term ventilation. Other muscle weaknesses may also result from the disease. Affected children may be unable to walk, swallow or use their hands. As the child ages, the affected limbs do not grow normally and look smaller ('withered').

For the child with polio, most difficulties are with mobility, fine motor activity and coordination. Attendant self-care difficulties may also occur.

The advice and considerations about the school environment curriculum and resources found under *Physical disability* will apply.

Useful links
Leicestershire Post-Polio Network
8 Heathgate Close
Birstall
Leicestershire LE4 3GU
Tel: 0116 220 9188
E-mail: helena.edwards@poliouk.org
http://beehive.thisisleicestershire.co.uk/
default.asp?WCI=SiteHome&ID=8147&Pa
geID=43630

The British Polio Fellowship
Eagle Office Centre
The Runway
South Ruislip
Middlesex HA4 6SE
Freephone: 0800 018 0586
E-mail: info@britishpolio.org
www.britishpolio.org/

Polyarthritis *see Arthritis*

Port-wine stain

Port-wine stain is also known as naevus
flammeus. It can occur on the head or face.
It does not disappear as the child ages and
can be a cause of teasing, bullying and
consequently low self-esteem. When associated with *Cerebral palsy* (Hemiplegia), *Epilepsy*
and learning difficulties, it is known as
Sturge–Weber syndrome. In this condition
there are abnormal blood vessels within the
brain. Laser treatments for the skin condition are available.

For some children their differences have
social and psychological effects. Staff in
school can do a number of things to help,
including watching for cruel taunts, playground unpleasantness, social avoidance and
withdrawal (see *Disfigurement and difference*).
Careful sympathetic support will go a long
way. Pupils who taunt and bully will need
attention consistent with school policy.
Some youngsters will avoid doing sport
because of the need to remove clothes in
changing rooms. In order to help children
understand and accept their differences, it is
important to work closely with parents/
carers.

The curriculum will not need to be modified for children because they have a
port-wine stain.

Useful links
Birthmark Support Group
PO Box 3932
Weymouth DT4 9YG
E-mail:
info@birthmarksupportgroup.org.uk
www.birthmarksupportgroup.org.uk

British Association of Dermatologists
19 Fitzroy Square
London W1T 6EH
Tel: 020 7383 0266
Fax: 020 7388 5263
E-mail: admin@bad.org.uk
www.skinhealth.co.uk/contact/index.htm

Prader–Willi syndrome

Prader–Willi syndrome is caused when the
child inherits faulty copies of part of chromosome 15 with loss of genetic material.
Affected children can have low muscle tone,
obsession with food and eating, obesity, and

learning and behavioural difficulties. Many children later on develop diabetes and skin infections.

Problems can relate to eating behaviours and a preoccupation with food. Later on learning problems and diabetes might contribute further to the child's difficulty in learning effectively.

Children with Prader–Willi syndrome will have their needs met in a range of mainstream and special schools. Some children will need a small amount of support and guidance in their lives while others need constant attention.

Good communication between home and school is very important. Effective school-based *Interdisciplinary working* is necessary and may possibly include health visitors, educational psychologists and dieticians. A team approach is necessary to design programmes to address the child's drive to satisfy an insatiable appetite. Good pastoral systems are necessary and staff will need to consider how they are going to manage food-related events such as school parties, break-time snacks, food technology lessons and lunch times. Careful planning and thought can provide the child with a supportive learning environment with carefully planned access to food.

Some children show very difficult obsessive and compulsive behaviours that can be trying in a classroom, so strategies for withdrawal to a different teaching area might be needed. Some children can show extreme behaviours including physical violence and self-mutilation and, in these cases, physical interventions by suitably trained and experienced staff will be necessary. Many children need a carefully designed behaviour management plan, agreed with parents and systematically applied throughout the school day.

Careful attention to communication will be needed as many children have poor auditory skills and might not be able to manage too many instructions at the same time. It is helpful to keep things as simple as possible using visual aids and careful but insistent requests. Some children will show great inflexibility and need to repeat or question things persistently – great patience will be needed by staff and peers. Some children can find unplanned changes to routine events difficult to manage, so it is important to develop a means for the child to deal with unplanned changes. One strategy is to consistently use a special form of words that reassure. It can also help to use a special place for 'special communications' about unplanned change. Overall children with Prader–Willi syndrome have a condition that will to some extent affect their education.

Useful links
The Prader–Willi Syndrome Association (UK)
33 Leopold Street
Derby DE1 2HF
Tel: 01332 365676
www.pwsa-uk.demon.co.uk

Prophylactic antibiotics

Prophylactic antibiotics are antibiotics given to prevent infections from taking hold and are often given to children with immune problems, chronic chest disorders (not asthma), and urinary or kidney problems.

The administration of these medications is unlikely to need to take place at school.

Pseudohypoparathyroidism *see* Hypoparathyroidism

Psoriasis

Psoriasis is a chronic skin condition that is relatively rare in childhood. It causes inflammation with redness, dryness and flakiness of the skin. Sometimes the skin condition is accompanied by arthritis. The nails can also be affected. Treatment is generally with steroid creams and with moisturisers to reduce itching.

Children with psoriasis can be educated in mainstream and special schools. The extent to which psoriasis affects schooling depends on the medical interventions required and most children will have their condition managed by community medical services. Effective links with parents and good pastoral arrangements will provide the child with support.

Children with psoriasis will not need modifications to the curriculum. Staff should be aware of the supportive things they can do in the event of a problem. Most children are knowledgeable about the ways to manage their treatment but might need support with some dressings. Special arrangements for swimming will probably be needed where skin needs treatment.

Useful links
The Psoriasis Association
7 Milton Street
Northampton NN2 7JG

Tel: 01604 711129
E-mail: mail@psoriasis.demon.co.uk
www.timewarp.demon.co.uk/psoriasis.html

Psoriatic arthritis *see* Arthritis

Ptosis *see* Treacher Collins syndrome

Pulmonary atresia

Pulmonary atresia is a form of congenital heart defect where the right side of the heart and the artery from the heart to the lungs do not form properly, leading to an inability of the heart to pump blood to the lungs to be re-oxygenated. It leads to the newborn baby being blue. Early treatment involves an operation to allow more blood to pump through the lungs. Later treatment involves a series of operations to attempt to allow the blood returning from the body to flow directly through the lungs (without the heart having to pump it through) and to let the left ventricle pump the oxygenated blood around the body (the Fontan Procedure). Children with these problems may find it hard to take part in physical exercise. See *Congenital heart diseases*.

Pulmonary stenosis

Pulmonary stenosis is a congenital heart defect where the flow of blood from the right side of the heart to the lungs (where blood is oxygenated) is restricted because of a narrowing of the pulmonary valve. Severe cases will cause symptoms in the newborn, while milder defects might only cause breathlessness in older children. Treatment is to widen the narrowing with a special balloon introduced into the heart via a special flexible tube, called a catheter. For the child at school, the main impact of a significant narrowing will be on their ability to take part in strenuous physical exercise (see *Congenital heart diseases*).

Pyelonephritis *see* Urinary tract infection

R

Reactive arthritis

Reactive arthritis is a swelling of a joint or joints that occurs following an earlier infection (for example, a sore throat). The child can experience pain, swelling and loss of joint function. This in turn can affect mobility, manipulation and self-care. Treatment is to try and reduce pain and swelling.

Children with reactive arthritis can be educated in mainstream and special schools. The extent to which this condition affects schooling depends on severity and the medical interventions required. For some children pain management is important; others might experience periods of restricted mobility and will need exercises designed by a physiotherapist. School-based *Interdisciplinary working* involving a physiotherapist and an occupational therapist might be necessary for some children, while others will have their condition managed by community medical services. Effective links with parents and good pastoral arrangements will provide the child with support.

Children with arthritis will need access to the same curriculum as their peers. Children in the primary phase may need special attention; they might not tell staff when there is discomfort or a problem because they are engrossed in a particular activity or because they might prefer to avoid treatment. Some children will need wheelchairs; therefore access to classrooms and the building needs to be good (see *Physical disability*). The advice of medical professionals might be needed to ensure that exercises, activities and games in

PE are appropriate. Overall children with reactive arthritis have a condition, usually temporary, that can sometimes interfere with their education.

Useful links
Arthritis Care Youth Service
The Source
18 Stephenson Way
London NW1 2HD
Tel: 0808 808 2000
E-mail: thesource@arthritiscare.org.uk
www.arthritiscare.org.uk

Children's Chronic Arthritis Association
Ground Floor Office, Amber Gate
City Walls Road
Worcester WR1 2AH
Tel: 01905 745595

Reflux nephropathy *see* Vesicoureteric reflux

Refractive error

Refractive error (myopia, hypermetropia) means the lens of the eye cannot focus light exactly at the back of the eye. When the lens focuses light in front of the retina, the eye is shortsighted, or myopic. When the opposite happens (light focused behind the retina), the eye is longsighted (hypermetropic). Once diagnosed, treatment is with corrective lenses. Undiagnosed children will have difficulty accessing visual information.

Children with refractive errors can experience eyestrain and headache. The large majority of children with refractive errors will need to wear spectacles. Younger children should be encouraged to look after their spectacles and keep them clean. Children with refractive errors can be educated mainly in mainstream schools. Staff should be aware of the possible consequences of eyestrain and balance work accordingly. The curriculum will not need to be modified for children because they have refractive errors.

Useful links
Hands and Eyes
A USA specialist teacher maintains this useful online newsletter for teachers and caregivers of visually impaired students and their friends. It includes art, cooking and manipulative activities that visually impaired students can do individually or in small groups. It is for teachers and support staff in need of ideas for classroom activities and is particularly useful for pupils with multiple impairments such as developmental disability and motor impairment.
www.home.earthlink.net/~vharris/

RNIB Education Information Services
224 Great Portland Street
London W1N 6AA
Tel: 020 7388 1266
E-mail: webmaster@rnib.org.uk
www.rnib.org.uk
RNIB's curriculum information service offers information and advice to all professionals supporting a visually impaired child in mainstream or special schools.
www.rnib.org.uk/curriculum/
RNIB's accessing technology pages provide information about applications of technology in employment, at study and in leisure.
www.rnib.org.uk/technology/

V.I. Guide
This site contains information on many topics relating to parenting and teaching a child with visual impairments.
www.viguide.com/

Renal dialysis

Renal dialysis is a technique for replacing the normal function of a failing kidney. There are two main methods. In haemodialysis, the child's blood is pumped through special membranes; on the other side of the membranes are special salt solutions that allow impurities from the blood and unwanted salts and fluid to cross the membrane and thus be removed. The technique takes time and has to be repeated several times a week; this can prove highly disruptive to a child. In chronic ambulatory peritoneal dialysis, the special salt solutions are introduced into the abdomen and the body's own peritoneal membrane is used to allow the impurities, waste products and unwanted salts and fluid to pass into the solution, which is then removed. This again takes time and has to be repeated several times a week. A successful renal transplant with a healthy kidney can restore normal renal function to the child and result in a return to a much more normal quality of life, although drugs will be needed to prevent rejection of the transplanted kidney. Renal failure that requires these techniques produces severe psychological disruption for the child, failure to grow and gain weight properly, and, in older children, a failure to enter puberty at the normal time.

Children requiring renal dialysis can be educated in mainstream and special schools. The extent to which treatment affects schooling depends on the arrangements for dialysis. School-based *Interdisciplinary working* might be helpful for some children, while others will have their condition managed by community medical services. Effective links with parents and good pastoral arrangements will provide the child with support.

Children requiring renal dialysis will be learning to manage their time and will probably be receiving the support of teachers working for the local hospital school. Links between school and hospital school need to be strong and effective in order to maintain continuity and consistency across the curriculum.

Overall, children having renal dialysis must be regarded as children who have a condition that will affect their education.

Useful links
National Kidney Federation
6 Stanley Street
Worksop S81 7HX
Tel: 0845 601 0209
E-mail: helpline@kidney.org.uk
www.kidney.org.uk

Nephronline
E-mail: info@nephronline.org
www.nephronline.org/

Restricted growth *see* Short stature

Retinitis pigmentosa

Retinitis pigmentosa is a progressive condi-tion where the light-sensitive pigment layer at the back of the eye gradually degenerates, leading to increasing visual loss. The condition can first show itself as night-blindness, although later on there is progressive loss of the peripheral vision. Macular dystrophy is a similar type of disease, although, here, the central part of the retina is affected first. This leads to rapidly reduced vision, although the condition can eventually stabilise with some residual vision remaining.

Children with deteriorating vision can be educated in mainstream and special schools. School-based *Interdisciplinary working*, including the advice of a specialist teacher for visual impairment, will be necessary for some children, while community medical services will manage others. Children who have deteriorating vision will experience a loss of sight that varies according to different factors. Some children will have tunnel vision and will be able to make good use of residual vision, while others will experience severe visual impairment. Enlarging print size does not solve the problem for all types of retinitis pigmentosa. If a child has a narrow field of vision, then it can be more helpful to keep the print at a normal size to maximise the numbers of words that they can see, but reading can be aided by printing the letters in 'bold' type. Lighting levels and angles of light can be very important to the pupil with retinitis pigmentosa. Both the child and the advisory teacher for the visually impaired should be consulted on the best position, levels and control of lighting. For further advice see *Visual impairment* or *Blindness*. Generally children with a deteriorating retina will need adaptations to the curriculum (see *Usher syndrome*).

Useful links
Hands and Eyes

A USA specialist teacher maintains this useful online newsletter for teachers and caregivers of visually impaired students and their friends. It includes art, cooking and manipulative activities that visually impaired students can do individually or in small groups. It is for teachers and support staff in need of ideas for classroom activities and is particularly useful for pupils with multiple impairments such as developmental disability and motor impairment.
www.home.earthlink.net/~vharris/

Retinitis Pigmentosa Society
PO Box 350
Buckingham MK18 5EL
Tel: 01280 860363
www.brps.demon.co.uk

RNIB Education Information Services
224 Great Portland Street
London W1N 6AA
Tel: 020 7388 1266
E-mail: webmaster@rnib.org.uk
www.rnib.org.uk
RNIB's curriculum information service offers information and advice to all professionals supporting a visually impaired child in mainstream or special schools.
www.rnib.org.uk/curriculum/
RNIB's accessing technology pages provide information about applications of technology in employment, at study and in leisure.
www.rnib.org.uk/technology/

V.I. Guide
This site contains information on many topics relating to parenting and teaching a child with visual impairments.
www.viguide.com/

Retinoblastoma

Retinoblastoma is a malignant tumour of the eye found in children. For further advice see *Cancer*. It sometimes runs in families and can affect both eyes. If caught early enough, the condition is curable with radiotherapy. The condition can also be treated by surgical removal of the affected eye. These children may have minor visual loss or be completely blind in one or both eyes depending on the stage of the tumour, whether both eyes are affected and on the treatment offered. Children with retinoblastoma might retain one eye with good vision and many are able to retain the use of both eyes; they live normal lives but need care and attention for the duration of their treatment.

Children with retinoblastoma can be educated in mainstream and special schools. School-based *Interdisciplinary working* might be necessary for some children, while others will have their condition managed by the appropriate medical services. Games such as squash, badminton and some contact sports that could damage the remaining eye should be avoided. For children with both eyes affected, there is likely to be more significant impairment (see *Visual impairment*).

Useful links
Hands and Eyes

A USA specialist teacher maintains this useful online newsletter for teachers and caregivers of visually impaired students and their friends. It includes art, cooking and manipulative activities that visually impaired students can do individually or in small groups. It is for teachers and support staff in need of ideas for classroom activities and is particularly useful for pupils with multiple impairments such as

developmental disability and motor impairment.
www.home.earthlink.net/~vharris/

Retinoblastoma Society
St Bartholomew's Hospital
West Smithfield
London EC1A 7BE
Tel: 020 7600 3309
E-mail: rbinfo@rbsociety.org.uk
www.retinoblastoma.com/

RNIB Education Information Services
224 Great Portland Street
London W1N 6AA
Tel: 020 7388 1266
E-mail: webmaster@rnib.org.uk
www.rnib.org.uk
RNIB's curriculum information service offers information and advice to all professionals supporting a visually impaired child in mainstream or special schools.
www.rnib.org.uk/curriculum/
RNIB's accessing technology pages provide information about applications of technology in employment, at study and in leisure.
www.rnib.org.uk/technology/

V.I. Guide
This site contains information on many topics relating to parenting and teaching a child with visual impairments.
www.viguide.com/

Retinopathy of prematurity

Retinopathy of prematurity (ROP) occurs in babies who were born at least two months early. It is a condition caused by the abnormal development of blood vessels at the back of the eye, leading to retinal detachment and scarring at the back of the eye. In school-aged children, it will be the effects of this condition on vision that will be seen. The condition can be treated, although some children may still experience varying degrees of visual loss. As it occurs in very premature infants, some of these children will also have other difficulties resulting from their early birth.

Children with ROP can be educated in mainstream and special schools. School-based *Interdisciplinary working* including the advice of a specialist teacher for visual impairment might be necessary for some children, while community medical services will manage others. For further advice see *Visual impairment* and *Blindness*.

Children with ROP usually develop normal central vision. Some children might have late complications, including strabismus (*Squint*, or crossed eyes), amblyopia ('lazy eye'), *Myopia* (short-sightedness) *Glaucoma* and late-onset retinal detachment.

Generally children with retinopathy of prematurity are likely to need some modification to the curriculum.

Useful links
Hands and Eyes
A USA specialist teacher maintains this useful online newsletter for teachers and caregivers of visually impaired students and their friends. It includes art, cooking and manipulative activities that visually impaired students can do individually or in small groups. It is for teachers and support staff in need of ideas for classroom activities and is particularly useful for pupils with multiple impairments such as developmental disability and motor impairment.
www.home.earthlink.net/~vharris/

RNIB Education Information Services
224 Great Portland Street
London W1N 6AA
Tel: 020 7388 1266
E-mail: webmaster@rnib.org.uk
www.rnib.org.uk
RNIB's curriculum information service offers information and advice to all professionals supporting a visually impaired child in mainstream or special schools.
www.rnib.org.uk/curriculum/
RNIB's accessing technology pages provide information about applications of technology in employment, at study and in leisure.
www.rnib.org.uk/technology/

V.I. Guide
This site contains information on many topics relating to parenting and teaching a child with visual impairments.
www.viguide.com/

Rett's syndrome

Rett's syndrome is a congenital condition seen only in girls, caused by a genetic defect. It manifests as developmental delay often not apparent during the first year of life but then becoming marked, leading to severe learning difficulties, restricted growth, *Scoliosis,* movement difficulties, a small head, abnormal breathing patterns and loss of useful hand function, although hand wringing movements are often seen. Many girls have *Epilepsy* and cold red feet, and grind their teeth.

On some occasions the condition might not be diagnosed for the first few years of life and may initially be confused with *Autism.* Diagnosis can be aided by performing an EEG recording. Genetic testing is available now. The progression of the condition with attendant loss of skills requires a developmental programme designed to maintain physical and mobility skills and abilities for as long as possible. The condition leads to life-long difficulties and dependency. Many girls will be profoundly and multiply disabled and require high levels of staffing. Hand wringing needs to be considered by a medical team and solutions, such as splints, can affect curriculum access and raise issues of restraint. Hyperventilation and breath-holding require vigilance from the class team. School-based *Interdisciplinary working* is crucial as well as counselling for parents.

Girls will usually require education in a single-storey building with good wheelchair access, including good-sized classrooms able to accommodate special equipment and sensory facilities. It is helpful to have access to sensory, soft play and hydrotherapy facilities. Accommodation for therapists to work and meet together with medical facilities is desirable.

These girls need a highly modified and developmental curriculum. The sensory curriculum is essential and any programme will need to include careful attention to monitoring a girl's skills and consolidating achievements to date. Class teams should develop detailed assessment, recording and reporting strategies in order to support the medical assessments that mark the progress of the condition. The motor skills component of the PE curriculum should include regular monitoring by a physiotherapist. There's a wide recognition that music and in particular music therapy is of great value.

Useful links
National Rett Syndrome Association
15 Tanzieknowe Drive
Glasgow G72 8RG
Tel: 0141 641 7662

Rett Syndrome Association UK
113 Friern Barnet Road
London N11 3EU
Tel: 020 8361 5161
E-mail: info@rettsyndrome.org.uk
www.rettsyndrome.org.uk

Rhinitis

Rhinitis literally means the inflammation of the nasal passages. It is usually the result of allergy to pollens, grasses and animal hair. It is most commonly seen in children with hay fever (who may also have red, sore and itchy eyes – vernal conjunctivitis – see *Conjunctivitis*) and causes a blocked or runny nose. Treatment is with nasal sprays and antihistamine medicines. The seasonal nature of hay fever means that some children are most adversely affected in the late spring and summer during examinations and assessments.

Children with rhinitis can be educated in mainstream and special schools. The extent to which rhinitis affects schooling depends on the severity of the condition and medical interventions required. This condition is usually simply managed by community medical services. Effective links with parents and good pastoral arrangements might be needed.

Children with rhinitis should not need different curriculum arrangements to their peers. Staff should be aware of the supportive things they can do in those circumstances that might exacerbate the condition; for example consideration of environmental factors and seasonal variables. Some families will want to explore diets excluding certain foods, and schools can help parents by managing access to permitted foods and supervising snacks at break times.

Useful links
Action against Allergy
PO Box 278
Twickenham TW1 4QQ
Tel: 020 8892 2711
E-mail:
AAA@actionagainstallergy.freeserve.co.uk
www.actionagainstallergy.co.uk

Breathe Easy
British Lung Foundation
78 Hatton Garden
London EC1N 8LD
Tel: 020 7831 5831
E-mail: blf@britishlungfoundation.com
www.lunguk.org

British Allergy Foundation
Deepdene House
30 Bellegrove Road
Welling DA16 3PY
Tel: 020 8303 8583
E-mail: info@allergyfoundation.com
www.allergyfoundation.com

National Society for Research into Allergies and Environmental Diseases
PO Box 45

Hinckley LE10 1JY
Tel/Fax: 01455 250715
E-mail: nsra.allergy@virgin.net

Rickets

Rickets is a condition that tends to affect younger children and results in soft bones. It is caused by a lack of vitamin D. This can lead to mobility problems, but it is now rare in the UK.

Useful links
XLH Network
Elpha Green Cottage
Sparty Lea
Allendale
Hexham NE47 9UT
Tel: 01434 685047
E-mail: Larry.Winger@ncl.ac.uk
http://xlhnetwork.ncl.ac.uk

S

Sanfillipo syndrome *see* Mucopolysaccharidosis

Scabies

Scabies is caused by a mite that burrows under the skin. It causes a very itchy rash that may become infected after prolonged scratching. It is usual to treat the whole family at once to avoid re-infection. Treatment is with a skin lotion that kills the mite. The child can remain itchy once the mite has been killed, although by then the risk of infestation will no longer be present.

It is unusual for children to get scabies; however, it can break out in school and will need treating as recommended by community healthcare teams. Pupils with scabies should not be in school until 24 hours after treatment has been completed. It is normal practice to notify parents of children who may have had direct contact with the infected child. A school generally needs to work alongside health colleagues to promote awareness, eradicate the stigma, identify infestations and teach children good healthcare habits. In some situations children and families will need support and counselling.

The curriculum will not need to be modified for children because they have scabies.

Useful links
British Association of Dermatologists
19 Fitzroy Square
London W1T 6EH
Tel: 020 7383 0266

Fax: 020 7388 5263
E-mail: admin@bad.org.uk
www.skinhealth.co.uk/contact/index.htm

School phobia

School phobia describes children who refuse to go to, or are fearful of attending, school because of educational, social or emotional reasons. They prefer to stay with their carers who are aware of their absence from school – this is therefore not truancy. Children are usually fearful and anxious and exhibit symptoms related to their feelings.

Any significant stress, trauma, anxiety or condition can trigger avoidance of school. Where possible school staff will need to work closely with parents and carers to identify the root cause of school avoidance. Once a cause has been established, it may be possible to begin to work with the child to address the problem by reintroducing him or her to school gradually. In extreme cases the support of external professionals, such as counsellors, an educational psychologist, education welfare officer, and psychiatric nurse might be needed (see *Interdisciplinary working*). Re-integration into the school environment is usually the most effective intervention.

It is very important for the school to have excellent pastoral systems in order to provide the child with reassurance and nurture during their most anxious periods. It is helpful to create stable structures and actively encourage positive and supportive friendships.

Class work needs to be achievable and not overdemanding; homework needs to be interesting and exciting so that parents/carers are able to focus on very real positives about the school.

School refusal syndrome *see* School phobia

Scoliosis

Scoliosis is the term applied to abnormal bends in the spine. It can occur as an isolated condition in otherwise healthy children or as part of a neuromuscular condition, for example *Duchenne muscular dystrophy*. Treatment of a slight bend could be with a brace, although more severe cases may require surgery to straighten the spine. The deformity caused by scoliosis might pose problems for the child. Advanced scoliosis can adversely affect the child's breathing.

Children with scoliosis can be educated in mainstream and special schools. The extent to which this condition affects schooling depends on medical interventions. School-based *Interdisciplinary working* involving a physiotherapist and an occupational therapist might be necessary for some children, while others will have their condition managed by community medical services. Effective links with parents and good pastoral arrangements will provide the child with support.

Children with scoliosis will need access to the same curriculum as their peers. The advice of medical professionals might be needed to ensure that exercises, activities and games in PE are appropriate.

Useful links
Scoliosis Association (UK)

2 Ivebury Court
325 Latimer Road
London W10 6RA
Tel: 020 8964 1166
E-mail: info@sauk.org.uk
www.sauk.org.uk

Sensorineural hearing loss

Sensorineural hearing loss is sometimes known as nerve deafness. The nerve that transmits the impulses generated by the ear in response to sound waves fails to work properly. Some children are born with nerves that did not form properly (congenital sensorineural deafness) while in others the nerve is damaged by trauma, toxins, drugs or infection. The implications for the child's hearing and access to the curriculum are similar whatever the cause of the problem, although congenital nerve deafness will by definition affect the child's ability to learn speech.

The impact on a child's education and learning language can be significant; the advice found under *Hearing impairment* will apply. An effective means of communication is central to providing special education for children with sensorineural hearing loss. Some children might benefit from a *Hearing aid* to hear and understand language, while others could use one for more basic purposes such as being alerted to sounds.

Children with sensorineural hearing loss can be educated in mainstream and special schools. School-based *Interdisciplinary working* involving specialist teachers, audiologists and audio technicians might be necessary for some children, while community medical services will manage others. Effective links with parents and good pastoral arrangements will provide support for these children.

Attention to language acquisition and communication will be vital. The child who has lost hearing prelingually (became deaf before acquiring language) and a child who has lost hearing postlingually (became deaf after exposure to and acquisition of language) will have different requirements in terms of speech and language development. Teachers will need to work very closely with the speech and language therapist in order to provide the differentiated communication required.

Separation anxiety disorder

Separation anxiety disorder is when a child refuses to attend school because of abnormally high anxiety at being separated from parents/carers – see *School phobia*. The assistance of a skilled child counsellor and psychiatrist are usually required (see *Interdisciplinary working*). With care the academic requirements of the curriculum can be maintained during treatment through homework and the involvement of outreach teachers. A graduated and extended transition plan can provide a child with support in returning to school.

Septic arthritis *see* Osteomyelitis

Sexually transmitted diseases

Sexually transmitted diseases include herpes virus infections, anogenital warts, chlamydial infections, gonorrhoea, syphilis, hepatitis B (see *Hepatitis*) and HIV/AIDS (see *Human immunodeficiency virus*). All young people who are old enough to be sexually active are potentially at risk through sexual relationships, and children of all ages are potentially at risk from sexual abuse.

Children infected by sexually transmitted diseases can be educated in mainstream and special schools. Most children will have their condition managed by community medical services. Effective links with parents and good pastoral arrangements will provide the child with support.

The school will have a sex education policy that will outline the school's curriculum including how children are to be taught about sexually transmitted diseases (see *Human immunodeficiency virus*). It is unlikely that the curriculum should be modified for children because they have a sexually transmitted disease.

Useful links
Sheffield Centre for HIV & Sexual Health
22 Collegiate Crescent
Sheffield S10 2BA
Tel: 0114 226 1900
E-mail: chiv.admin@chs.nhs.uk
www.sexualhealthsheffield.co.uk

Society of Health Advisers in Sexually Transmitted Diseases
MSF Centre
33–37 Moreland Street
London EC1V 8BB
E-mail: Martin.Murchie@glacomen.scot.nhs.uk
www.shastd.org.uk

Short stature

Short stature can be due to a variety of reasons. In some children this is because they are 'programmed' to grow and physically develop at a slow pace (but at a normal rate). Some might be related to nutritional problems, for example *Crohn's disease*, or the side effects of drug therapy (renal disease requiring high-dose, long-term steroids), emotional neglect and abuse, hormone deficiencies (such as *Hypothyroidism* or growth hormone deficiency – see *Growth hormone*) or genetic syndromes (*Achondroplasia*, *Down's syndrome*) that cause restricted growth.

Children with restricted growth can be educated in mainstream and special schools. School-based *Interdisciplinary working* involving an occupational therapist might be necessary for some children, while community medical services will manage others. Effective links with parents and good pastoral arrangements will provide the child with support.

The educational arrangements for children with short stature will vary widely between individuals and be largely dependant on the cause. A modified curriculum will be required for some children. Adaptations will need to compensate when necessary for impaired motor activity and occasionally mobility. An individual educational programme should be designed to include movement skills, self-help and independence skills, and social and daily living skills (see *Physical disability*, *Mucopolysaccharidosis* and *Turner's syndrome*). The advice of medical professionals might be needed to ensure that exercises, activities and games in PE are appropriate. Some children could be bullied and teased at school and adults who are not informed might make false assumptions about their age. These and other unhelpful experiences could impact negatively on their self-esteem (see *Disfigurement and difference*).

Useful links
Bone Dysplasia Group
c/o Child Growth Foundation
2 Mightfield Avenue
Chiswick
London W4 1PW
Tel: 020 8994 7625

Child Growth Foundation
2 Mightfield Avenue
Chiswick
London W4 1PW
Tel: 020 8994 7625

Restricted Growth Association
PO Box 4744
Dorchester DT2 9FA
Tel: 01308 898445
E-mail: rga1@talk21.com
www.rgaonline.org.uk

Sickle cell anaemia

Sickle cell anaemia is caused by having an abnormal sort of haemoglobin in the blood (see *Anaemia*). This results in the red blood cells clumping together during infections, periods of strenuous exercise or dehydration. As the cells clump together, they block off small blood vessels causing severe pain (painful crises) and other problems, such as anaemia, infections and possible restricted growth.

Children with sickle cell anaemia can be

educated in mainstream and special schools. School-based *Interdisciplinary working* might be necessary for some children, while community medical services will manage others. Children with sickle cell anaemia will need access to the same curriculum as their peers, although they might present as under-achievers because of absence from school. Some children experience frequent periods of illness together with courses of treat-ment. Frequent absence from schoo can lead to staff having low expectations of chil-dren's achievements and school friendships will be disrupted. It is important to explore all possible ways of supporting children who are regularly absent and to provide a range of ways to help them catch up with work; this becomes very important where children are mid-syllabus for externally accredited exami-nations. It is important to make sure that children can drink plenty of fluids through-out the school day. It is unlikely that the curriculum should be modified for children because they have sickle cell anaemia.

Useful links
Organisation for Sickle Cell Anaemia Research (OSCAR)
5 Lauderdale House
Cowley Estate
London SW9 6JS
Tel: 020 7735 4166

The Sickle Cell Society
54 Station Road
London NW10 4UA
Tel: 020 8961 7795/4006
E-mail: sicklecellsoc@btInternet.com
www.sicklecellsociety.org

Slipped femoral epiphysis

Slipped femoral epiphysis affects the hips and is caused by movement of the growing bone just beneath the head of the thigh bone. It is more common in boys (usually in later childhood) and causes pain in either hip or knee, and can lead to immobility or diffi-culty walking. Surgery is sometimes required.

The advice and considerations about the school environment, curriculum and resources found under *Physical disability* will apply. It is unlikely that the curriculum will need to be modified for children because they have slipped femoral epiphysis; however some children will be absent from school whilst receiving treatment.

Useful links
STEPS
Lymm Court
11 Eagle Brow
Lymm WA13 0LP
Tel: 01925 757525
E-mail: info@steps-charity.org.uk
www.steps-charity.org.uk/

Sly syndrome *see* Mucopolysaccharidosis

Smith–Magenis syndrome

Smith–Magenis syndrome is a rare condition caused by the loss of genetic material from chromosome 17. It can cause problems with abnormal facial features (a flattened middle part of the face and down-turned mouth), growth, feeding, *Epilepsy*, speech and language, hearing and learning. Learning difficulties are often severe. It also causes sleep disturbance, behavioural difficulties and self-mutilation (e.g. biting). Some affected children also stick beads and other objects into their noses and ears.

Children with this condition will have a wide range of needs at school and these will be complicated by the attendant behavioural difficulties that go along with the condition.

Children with Smith-Magenis syndrome can look different to other children (see *Disfigurement and difference*). Their physical condition and intellectual impairments generally require a specialised educational environment providing a highly differentiated curriculum. Good *Interdisciplinary working* is crucial as the ongoing advice of speech and language therapists, occupational therapists and physiotherapists will be needed in the design of a good educational programme (see *Physical disability* and *Speech problems*).

Many children will have behavioural problems including hyperactivity, head banging, self-biting and other self-mutilating practices. With many children a carefully designed behaviour management plan should be systematically applied throughout the school day. These children will need high levels of support in all curriculum subjects and at all times during the school day.

Useful links
Smith–Magenis Syndrome Contact Group
42 Blackmore Rd
Malvern WR14 1QT
Tel: 01684 566606
or
52 Ladeside Close
Newton Mearns
Glasgow G77 6TZ

Specific learning difficulties – generic advice only

Children with specific learning difficulty will need an individualised educational programme designed to support their learning and minimise the impact of the difficulty. Because children with a specific learning difficulty make progress in other areas of learning, they will need targeted support and assistance that will enable them to keep up with their peers in the particular area(s) affected. Over time the specific problem will become evident to a child's classmates and care and support through the school's pastoral systems will be necessary to give positive signals about the child and his or her work, and to counter any unreasonable name calling or mistreatment resulting from the difficulty.

Specific learning difficulties include *Dyscalculia*, *Dyslexia*, *Dysgraphia*, *Attention deficit hyperactivity disorder (ADHD)* and *Minimal brain dysfunction*. There are many strategies for addressing children's learning and some very specialised programmes requiring strict regimes. It is beyond the scope of this entry to provide detailed information on programmes and approaches.

Curriculum plans and educational programmes will need designing and/or modifying to provide access, and good monitoring will be needed in order to identify the most effective ways in which the child is motivated and learns. The ways in which children can be helped depends on the specific difficulty. Early identification and a programme of strategies designed to give the child alternative routes to work successfully is required. Close attention to the mechanics of what needs to happen to support the child's learning can be very useful, for example where the child sits, the table and chair, holding of pencils and pens, organisation of resources and the materials that best suit the child. Multisensory approaches to teaching have proved very successful for many children with specific learning difficulties; a frequently used approach is Visual, Auditory, Kinaesthetic, and Tactile (VAKT). A child reading will normally see, hear and say words; using a multisensory approach adds touch, movement and the possibility of dividing words up into easy to learn parts. There are some excellent software packages that provide strong visual images with sound and a touchscreen providing the kinaesthetic dimension. School-based *Interdisciplinary working* including the advice of specialist teachers might be useful in developing a multisensory programme.

For most children with specific learning difficulties the major barrier to learning can be motivation. Therefore staff will need to know the child well so that plans include those elements that will minimise the possibility of failure and dissatisfaction. It can be very helpful to engage the support of parents in preparing for new topics, subjects and ideas, particularly where new words or symbols are used.

For older pupils at KS3+4 schools make sure that all subject teachers know what suits the individual learning needs of the youngster. It is beneficial to work with students in determining their own learning styles and to encourage them to let staff responsible for teaching subjects know how they need the curriculum organised.

Speech and language problems

Speech and language sits at the heart of the educational process. Because all communication disorders can isolate individuals from their social and educational surroundings, it is essential to find appropriate timely intervention. Children might have language difficulties and or speech difficulties, the former being about grammar and the latter about the physical ability to utter sounds. Some speech and language problems are not linked to any other impairment or disability and are known as 'specific language difficulties' or 'specific language impairment'. Initial delay in speech and language or early problems with speech pattern can sometimes be associated with later difficulties in learning. When children have muscular disorders, hearing problems or developmental delays, their acquisition of speech, language and related skills is often affected.

Where children have difficulties they will be seen by speech and language therapists who provide therapy for the child; consult with the child's teacher about the most effective ways to aid the child's communication in the class setting, and work closely with the family to develop goals and techniques for effective therapy in class and at home. Good *Interdisciplinary working* between therapist and teacher and good links with home are crucial.

Local authorities provide specialist speech and language units, outreach services and schools. Many children with speech and language problems are educated in mainstream settings and consequently communicate with a range of adults with varieties of skills and knowledge. SENCOs need to work carefully to ensure that children and young people with speech and language problems are known and the problems understood by other staff. For obvious reasons this is likely to be more demanding in the secondary phase where many adults provide the curriculum. Most special schools will have well-developed language and communication policies and strategies and have arrangements for working alongside speech and language therapists. Skilled and experienced educationalists will use a child's ability to communicate as an early indicator of cognitive development.

Speech problems

The ability to speak depends in part on the movements of the mouth including tongue, lips and palate combined with controlled breathing. The motor skills associated with poor speech production will require physical exercises. At the earliest stages of development these exercises will be linked to eating and chewing. Children who are not eating hard foods that require chewing will have less strength and therefore less muscle tone in the mouth, tongue and lips. Work on articulation is skilled and might need to be quite specific; some speech and language therapists specialise in this area of work.

The advice and programmes devised by therapists and specialist teachers need to be carried out carefully. Regular and frequent monitoring of the child by the therapist or specialist teacher is very important in order to maintain progress and ensure that the strategies are effective.

Work on articulation is often associated with rhymes and verse that include the

appropriate emphasis. This kind of work is more easily built into the primary curriculum. As children grow older it is less easy to include this work in the timetable. Sensitivity and care are needed and it might be necessary to make separate arrangements for exercises. In secondary schools SENCOs will need to make best use of pastoral systems and whole-school staff meetings in order to establish consistent approaches and strategies.

A number of children will use signs, symbols and pictures to aid their communication. A smaller number will use *Alternative and augmentative communication* (AAC) such as speech output devices. In these cases it is important to work closely with the specialist support staff involved. As in all aspects of learning difficulty, it is crucial to develop and encourage self-esteem and motivation. Where children make progress and strive to achieve, they need clear positive signals giving value to their efforts. It is important that the positive approach is adopted and integrated into the informal aspects of a school's life such as playtimes and school clubs.

Language delay or impairment

The acquisition of language is complex and the subject of research and debate. Recent dynamic research on brain activity is beginning to explain how language is learned. Spoken language is the combination of a number of skills including:

- motor skills – the physical requirements for speech as above
- phonology – the sounds that build into words and language

- intonation and cadence (stress) – the music of spoken language
- grammar – the combinations of words and parts of words to make phrases and sentences
- semantics – the meanings of words
- pragmatics – the ways in which language is used in certain contexts and how emotions/feelings are expressed.

Language is usually attained developmentally. It is very useful for teachers to have a good understanding of how children attain language and an appreciation of how the use of language is linked to learning. The development of reception – listening and reading – interacts inevitably with the development of expression – speaking and writing. A delay in language development will have implications for a child's cognitive, social and emotional development and can significantly affect their interactions and therefore self-esteem.

Teachers will need to decide with specialist professionals on the content of a programme designed to address language development. Some problems are very specific and this will determine the strategy to be adopted. For example, the approach for a hearing-impaired child will be linked to overcoming the hearing loss in all settings, whereas a child with *Dyspraxia* might struggle with the sequence and pattern of what is needed to produce coherent words in the right order.

It is very important that teachers carefully differentiate their language in their lessons so that children can have the access that they need to the lesson content; similarly teachers should be 'tuned' into the particular style or differences the child might have in expression.

Children with speech impairments will need encouragement and support across the curriculum particularly where technical language is introduced. For example where children have semantic and pragmatic disorders, then it might be necessary to provide intensive support, for topics or parts of the syllabus that depend on new words.

Some children should be taught language systematically and this usually requires withdrawal or small group work by specialists. Strategies used such as Hanen Early Language Intervention and WILSTAAR are designed for very young children, but might usefully be extended into statutory education. These programmes are generally for use by parents with the preschool child and include components such as interaction to promote social communication, pretend play, emergent literacy, peer interaction and the use of specific word targets that are reinforced by modelling and frequent repetition.

Useful links

Afasic
2nd Floor, 50–52 Great Sutton Street
London EC1V 0DJ
Tel: 020 7490 9410
E-mail: info@afasic.org.uk
www.afasic.org.uk

Hanen Programme
The Hanen Centre
Suite 403 – 1075 Bay Street
Toronto
Ontario M5S 2B1
Canada
Tel: 001 416 921 1073
www.hanen.org

I-CAN
4 Dyer's Buildings
Holborn
London EC1N 2QP
Tel: 0870 010 4066
E-mail: info@ican.org.uk
www.ican.org.uk

Speech delay

Children with speech delay need to be positively encouraged and developed in their communication skills. The advice in *Speech and language problems* will apply.

It is particularly important to develop good teaching and learning styles, to get to know a child well in order to pick up on their own subtle cues and to help them in the way that suits them best.

Close and effective working with a speech and language therapist is very important. It is useful to have an understanding of speech and language development as this will help with determining next steps.

Speech disorder

Speech is linked with a complicated interaction of sensory, motor, emotional and social communicative functions. Experience shows that it is becoming increasingly difficult to separate out speech disorders from other associated disabilities. Where complex speech disorders are involved, increased difficulties with reading and writing are common.

Speech impediments include a large number of conditions that can affect one or more areas of comprehension or expression.

Impairments can range from slight pronunciation difficulties to the severest central organic speech disorders. Speech disorders are often closely connected with other forms of disability.

Speech disorders can be grouped as follows:

- language development disorders
- problems with phonation
- problems with forming concepts, limited vocabulary
- problems with grammar.

These are generally confined to preschool and primary school children. Symptoms of language development problems in older children and young people are usually due to other conditions involving cognitive functions that might affect speaking and writing.

Disorders of the ability to speak
Battarism Increasingly clumsy and rapid speech after involuntary repetition or mistakes of pronunciation

Logophobia The fear of speaking

Mutism A child's choice or inability to speak due to psychological factors (see *Elective mutism*)

Stuttering Spasmodic repetition of individual sounds, syllables and words – these usually start when children are very young, but they can be worse if they continue into the secondary phase where they might be compounded by psychosocial factors (see *Stammering* and *Dysfluency*)

Vocal and organic disorders and those originating in the central nervous system

Alexia Loss of a previously acquired ability to read in consequence of disease or injury to the brain and distinct from dyslexia

Aphasia Speech disorder originating in the central nervous system after language acquisition is complete; this can be caused by brain disease or physical damage to the brain damage from strokes, trauma, epilepsy or infectious disease

Dysarthria A general term for defective speaking, usually owing to slurring or poor articulation; it is often seen in children with cerebellar, peripheral motor or muscular defects

Dysarthrophonia Problems with speech production originating in the brain or elsewhere in the central nervous system, also affecting voice production, nasality and breathing it; might lead to excessive hoarseness, a high-pitched voice or squeaky voice quality

Dysglossia Physical malformation of peripheral speech organs present at birth or occurring in later life (e.g. paralysis, harelip or cleft palate)

Some children are unable to cope in mainstream schools because of their speech impairments, even though they have normal hearing and are of average or only slightly lower than average intelligence.

Communicative impairments are correspondingly diverse, and can originate from within the individual affected or from the reactions or prejudiced attitudes of others.

An individual's subjective impression of their communicative disorder (misunderstandings and rejection by the outside world) can be worse than the 'objective' severity of the disorder itself.

The large majority of speech disorders, from the slightest impediment to the severest disability, arise between the ages of three and ten. This has implications for teachers and class-based support staff and their teamwork; effective *Interdisciplinary working* is essential. Many children make good progress and are 'cured' by the time they reach puberty. Longer-lasting speech disorders usually occur as a symptom of a more general disorder.

Pastoral arrangements need to be first rate. Children and young people do not need negative reactions to their speech from the outside world as this can become the cause of anxiety and further aggravate the speech disorder. Positive relationships need to be fostered with peers. All staff should be made aware of the particular condition and its treatment and have a shared/consistent approach to inappropriate reactions from peers. In some circumstances it might be useful to have access to skilled counselling.

Speech disorder can result in communication frustration and not infrequently challenging behaviours.

Useful links
Afasic
2nd Floor, 50–52 Great Sutton Street
London EC1V 0DJ
Tel: 020 7490 9410
E-mail: info@afasic.org.uk
www.afasic.org.uk

I-CAN
4 Dyer's Buildings
Holborn
London EC1N 2QP
Tel: 0870 010 4066
E-mail: info@ican.org.uk
www.ican.org.uk

Spina bifida

Spina bifida is a congenital condition caused by the failure of the spinal cord and column to form completely early on in pregnancy. This causes weakness in the muscles which are normally supplied by the nerves from the affected part of the spine and below. The weakened muscles can in turn lead to immobility and orthopaedic problems with the legs, hips and spine. The sense of feeling in the affected parts of the body can also be reduced, leading to poor circulation and a propensity to get skin sores or ulcers. It can also cause abnormalities in the formation of the brain and lead to *Hydrocephalus* and, in some, *learning difficulties*. The muscles affected also often regulate the emptying of the bowel and bladder which can lead to damage to the gut and kidneys.

Although children with spina bifida may encounter a wide range of physical, perceptual, intellectual, nutritional and continence difficulties which threaten their potential for learning and independence, many needs can be met by timely input from physiotherapy, occupational therapy, speech and language therapy and medical, surgical and orthopaedic specialists.

Children with spina bifida will be educated in all types of schools depending on needs and the organisation of schools locally.

The advice and considerations found under *Physical disability* will apply. Interdisciplinary working and the timely involvement of therapists and the medical team are crucial.

Children with spina bifida and hydrocephalus are often gregarious and personable. They can show above average verbal skills, although the level of comprehension is limited. Most children who solely have spina bifida fall within the 'normal' range of intelligence.

Children may have perceptual problems including understanding pictures, discriminating between shapes, recognising symbols, figure/ground discrimination, and spatial judgements (i.e. size, space, distance and direction). Impaired motor ability may involve dexterity of the hands and arms. They may have difficulty with writing implements, scissors and other equipment; left- and mixed-handedness is more common, with a possible delay in choosing a dominant hand. Encourage children to practise making letters and numerals using any medium that works for them.

Impaired perceptual and motor ability may lead to clumsiness and slow, untidy handwriting. This may upset some children, particularly if they fall behind in work and find it difficult to complete tasks on time. Look for exercise books with prominent lines and find special pencils and pens. Provide and value word processing and possibly speech-activated software and ensure children have sufficient time for work. Network with colleagues to find the best-adapted equipment. Impaired perceptual and motor ability is likely to impede the child's ability to draw, produce detailed diagrams and do map work. This may become an issue at higher levels in some subjects.

Children with spina bifida and hydrocephalus can be easily distracted at times and are often referred to as 'hyperactive' or having 'poor concentration'. This can decline as they become older, and some children become passive and lack interest and motivation. Try to give children individual attention and encourage work in small groups. Sit them near the front of the class, near to the teacher, and take care to spread workloads.

Tiredness and difficulty with understanding can lead to a child seeming inattentive or restless. Remind the child of the learning objective of the session, provide materials of interest and relevance and expect the child to stay 'on task'. Help children to develop their own system of monitoring themselves and make it possible for appropriate support to be unobtrusively available.

Children with spina bifida and hydrocephalus often have extensive vocabularies and appear to have no trouble understanding single words although some find difficulty with language for written work and expressing themselves. Children who appear to have slow thinking and comprehension speed should be encouraged to take time. Large amounts of concentrated information should be kept to a minimum. Ensure that all coming into contact formally with the child implement the advice of the speech and language therapist. Differentiate the language of the classroom to match the child's comprehension. Give relevant instructions one at a time

and provide time to think about responses or contributions. Give the child confidence by giving prompts and additional information to encourage success at all times. Where possible relate communication and ideas to those things that the child knows or that are relevant to interests or personal experience.

Some children with spina bifida and hydrocephalus have poor short-term memory and difficulties with the storage and retrieval of information. Visual memory may be less reliable than auditory and so the use of spoken language is preferable when providing information. Try to build in patterns, routines and repetition to learning experiences, using props such as calendars, timetables, notes, lists and simple diaries. Encourage children to talk themselves through activities. Help develop strategies for learning using word association.

Many children with spina bifida and hydrocephalus experience difficulty generalising and transferring learning from one situation to another. Provide rich and plentiful opportunities to generalise learning and problem-solving strategies. It may be necessary to model and shape solutions from one situation to another, giving relevant explanations.

A child may find it difficult to define the essence of a problem, find strategies for resolution, choose a solution, act accordingly, or adapt where necessary. Establish a 'can do' approach by providing options rather than the right or wrong choice. Some children have difficulties with planning and organisation that arise from an impaired ability to know when and where to start. This can be in day-to-day tasks or in novel or unstructured situations. As children mature and the need for greater autonomy becomes more significant, they may have trouble organising themselves to meet the demands of adulthood.

A useful way of supporting organisational skills is to use colour coding for books and equipment. For example, History books and files could be covered in yellow and corresponding yellow stickers be put on timetables to indicate to the child to collect History items. A younger child may need to have one colour or pattern to identify everything required at school. Good clear timetables are important; use pictures, symbols and words and ensure there are copies in all useful places.

Encourage planning; show an appreciation for planning outlines for work or topics. It can be useful to support the child in presenting ideas for assignments to make sure they produce good work and raise self-esteem.

Maths is the subject most likely to cause difficulty because of problems with perception, attention, comprehension, memory and planning and organisation. Children can be supported in managing basic number concepts by breaking the required tasks into several small steps with frequent opportunities to practise. Some children have a capacity to rote learn facts and procedures. For them, translating mathematical ideas in to concrete examples may require help. It will be important to work carefully with sequencing, spatial orientation, patterns, predictions, visualisation, mental calculations, estimation and deduction. The school's implementation of the national numeracy strategy can be sufficiently flexible to provide the right support.

Useful links
International Federation for Hydrocephalus and Spina Bifida
Mrs Teresa Cole
2 Buzzard Close
Hartford
Huntingdon
Cambridgeshire P18 7XB
Tel: 01480 435 407
E-mail: teresac@nationwideisp.net
www.ifglobal.org

Association for Spina Bifida and Hydrocephalus
42 Park Road
Peterborough PE1 2UQ
Tel: 01733 555988
E-mail: postmaster@asbah.org
www.asbah.org/

Spinal muscular atrophy

Spinal muscular atrophy affects the nerves in the spinal cord causing progressive weakness of the muscles. It can affect either sex and in its severest form can cause death in the first year or so of life. Diagnosis can be made using genetic testing. Affected school-aged children have weakness of the muscles that may vary from virtually undetectable to severe. No cognitive problems accompany the disease, but in some individuals prolonged immobility may lead to stiffness of the joints, deformity of the spine (see *Scoliosis*) and breathing difficulties.

Most difficulties are with mobility, fine motor activity and coordination. Attendant self-care difficulties may also be present.

The advice and considerations about the school environment curriculum and resources found under *Physical disability* will apply.

Useful links
JTSMA
Elta House
Birmingham Road
Stratford upon Avon
Warwickshire CV37 0AQ
Tel: 01789 267520
E-mail: jennifer@jtsma.org.uk
www. jtsma.org.uk/index.html

Squint

Squint (strabismus) is the term applied when the two eyes do not look in the same direction. A variety of terms are used to describe the direction and variability of this problem. The eyes might have different degrees of long- or short-sightedness, or problems with overactive or underactive eye muscles. Severe untreated squints might lead to blindness in one eye. Treatments available are glasses, patching, eye drops and surgery.

Children with squints will need attention according to where they might be in the process of medical intervention. The aims of treatment of squint are to preserve or restore vision, straighten the eyes and restore binocular vision. Where corrective surgery is carried out, school-based *Interdisciplinary working* will be necessary; the advice of health professionals and of a specialist teacher for visual impairment may be needed in the planning of an effective educational programme. The school's pastoral arrange-ments should be good, as children with squints can become the target for name-calling such as 'cross-eyed', 'boss-eyed' or 'wall-eyed'. Most children with squints will need to wear spectacles and arrangements for support in looking after spectacles might be required. It is unlikely that the curriculum should be modified for children because they have squints.

Useful links
Hands and Eyes
A USA specialist teacher maintains this useful online newsletter for teachers and caregivers of visually impaired students and their friends. It includes art, cooking and manipulative activities that visually impaired students can do individually or in small groups. It is for teachers and support staff in need of ideas for classroom activities and is particularly useful for pupils with multiple impairments such as developmental disability and motor impairment.
www.home.earthlink.net/~vharris/

RNIB Education Information Services
224 Great Portland Street
London W1N 6AA
Tel: 020 7388 1266
E-mail: webmaster@rnib.org.uk
www.rnib.org.uk
RNIB's curriculum information service offers information and advice to all professionals supporting a visually impaired child in mainstream or special schools.
www.rnib.org.uk/curriculum/
RNIB's accessing technology pages provide information about applications of technology in employment, at study and in leisure.
www.rnib.org.uk/technology/

V.I. Guide
This site contains information on many topics relating to parenting and teaching a child with visual impairments.
www.viguide.com/

Stammering

Stammering is the spasmodic repetition of individual sounds, syllables and words. These usually start when children are very young; they can be worse if they continue into the secondary phase where they might be compounded by psychosocial factors.

School-based *Interdisciplinary working* including the advice of a speech and language therapist might be necessary for some children. Effective links with parents and good pastoral arrangements will provide the child with support.

Most strategies for supporting children are based on reducing pressure to communicate. Staff need to be calm, kind and approachable at all times. It is helpful to slow down the rate of talking to let the class know that there is sufficient time to speak rather than drawing attention to stammering. Use easily understood language and reduce the number of questions. Develop daily classroom routines such as reciting the days of the week or counting and singing or speaking familiar words with a verse and rhythm as in nursery rhymes or poetry. Get to know those things that are more likely to make a child stammer such as being hurried; being interrupted; competing; fear of the consequences of what's been said; expressing emotions; expressing complex ideas or using relatively new vocabulary and sentence structures. Where a particular situation or circumstance is causing problems seek alternative approaches. Where possible, link learning to a personal interest or hobby, as children then are more relaxed and tend to be more fluent. Reading strategies can help, giving the child a concrete means of tackling a new or difficult word.

It is unlikely that the curriculum should be modified for children because they stammer.

Useful links
The British Stammering Association
15 Old Ford Road
London E2 9PJ
Tel: 020 8983 1003
www.stammering.org/

The Michael Palin Centre for Stammering Children
Finsbury Health Centre
Pine Street
London EC1R 0LP
Tel: 020 7530 4238
E-mail: info@stammeringcentre.org
**www.stammeringcentre.org/feedback/cont
act.html**

Stevens–Johnson syndrome

Stevens–Johnson syndrome is a skin rash that involves the lips, mouth and other mucous membranes. It occurs after certain infections or in response to certain drugs. It is usually short lived. The rash itself is not infectious, although it might look quite dramatic (see *Erythema multiforme*).

Strabismus *see* **Squint**

Strawberry naevus

Strawberry naevus is a pink, raised, fleshy birthmark. It is caused by a knot of small blood vessels (capillaries) forming just under the skin. The mark often grows for the first one to two years of life before shrinking away; most disappear by five years.

For some children, their differences have social and psychological effects. Staff in school can do a number of things to help, including watching for cruel taunts, playground unpleasantness, social avoidance and withdrawal (see *Disfigurement and difference*). Careful sympathetic support will go a long way. Pupils that taunt and bully will need attention consistent with school policy. Some youngsters will avoid doing sport because of the need to remove clothes in changing rooms. In order to help children understand and accept their differences it is sensible to work closely with parents/carers.

The curriculum will not need to be modified for children because they have birthmarks.

Useful links
Birthmark Support Group
PO Box 3932
Weymouth DT4 9YG
E-mail:
info@birthmarksupportgroup.org.uk
www.birthmarksupportgroup.org.uk

British Association of Dermatologists
19 Fitzroy Square
London W1T 6EH

Tel: 020 7383 0266
Fax: 020 7388 5263
E-mail: admin@bad.org.uk
www.skinhealth.co.uk/contact/index.htm

Strokes *see* **Brain haemorrhage**

Sturge–Weber syndrome *see* **Port-wine stain**

Substance abuse

Substance abuse takes place where children use any of a wide variety of drugs and other psychoactive substances. Examples include alcohol, solvents, marijuana, amphetamines and heroin. In some children substance abuse can lead to physical, mental, social or economic problems. Substance abuse might result in health problems, personal problems, loss of motivation, addiction, strained family relationships, or social or economic problems.

The school's pastoral systems should be able to support the child. Staff will need to work with children to help them understand the inappropriateness of their actions and teach them social responsibility. The affects of substance abuse on the child's ability to work well in classrooms might be considerable at times. Irritability and extreme or poor behaviour are significant barriers to learning. Physical dependency and addiction will need careful attention and the support of other professionals. Care has to be taken in the ways in which the educational needs of children who are abusing substances and themselves are addressed, as the messages given by a school to its pupil population cannot afford to be interpreted as condoning substance abuse. Many education authorities have specialist teams of workers trained and skilled in working with children abusing substances.

Useful links
National Drug Prevention Alliance
PO Box 594
Slough SL1 1AA
E-mail: ndpa@drugprevent.org.uk
www.drugprevent.demon.co.uk

Subtelomeric deletions

Subtelomeric deletions occur in some children with otherwise unexplained learning and developmental difficulties. In these conditions, small amounts of genetic material are lost from the ends of the chromosomes (parts of the cell nucleus that contains the genetic blueprint of the individual). Many children will have other health-related problems such as *Epilepsy* or unusual physical appearance. The children experience problems dependant on the specific difficulties that the deletions cause.

Children with subtelomeric deletions can be educated in mainstream and special schools, dependant on the degree to which they are affected. School-based *Interdisciplinary working* will be necessary, including the advice of specialist teachers, speech and language therapists and possibly an educational psychologist. Some children have a very different appearance (see *Disfigurement and difference*). Other children will have a range of physical difficulties (see *Physical disability*).

Useful links
Unique – The Rare Chromosome Disorder Support Group
PO Box 2189
Caterham CR3 5GN
Tel: 01883 330766
E-mail: info@rarechromo.org
www.rarechromo.org

Syncope

Syncope is the medical term for fainting. It can occur from a variety of causes, and is most common in older children. It can occur after a child has been standing for a long time, after standing up from sitting or from lying down. It can also occur after prolonged fasting, for instance just before lunch time. Syncope can also follow a response to unpleasant stimuli. The child becomes pale and slumps down or falls to the ground. Unconsciousness usually lasts only a few seconds and the child recovers fairly quickly. In younger children, syncope can follow minor trauma such as bumps to the head or even with temper tantrums. This is sometimes known as pallid syncope or reflex anoxic seizure. These episodes can sometimes be confused with fits, but are rarely associated with the twitching usually seen in a fit. The cause of syncope might be related to temporarily low blood pressure, sudden changes in heart rate or a low blood sugar. For the child, fainting can lead to a loss of confidence if the problem is recurrent.

Children with syncope can be educated in mainstream and special schools. The extent to which syncope affects schooling depends on how children manage the symptoms of their condition and the medical interventions required. Some children will need to lie down and rest; others need to be looked after following a faint. School-based *Interdisciplinary working* might be necessary for some children, while community medical services will manage others. Effective links with parents and good pastoral arrangements will provide the child with physical and emotional support. Exercises and postural management designed by health professionals can help children manage their condition. Classmates should be appropriately informed of their condition, particularly when children are having episodes that cause them to faint.

Children with syncope will need access to the same curriculum as their peers. Staff should be aware of the supportive things that they can do in the event of a faint. A school needs good systems of support and opportunities for children to catch up after periods of absences. Special dietary arrangements will help some children, and regular access to food and drink is important. The advice of medical professionals might be needed to ensure that exercises, activities and games in PE are appropriate and will not aggravate the condition. It is usually important for children to take fluid before any physical activity. The safety measures for all pupils are generally sufficient.

Overall children with syncope must be regarded as children who happen to have a condition that will occasionally interfere with their education.

Useful links
Syncope Trust and Reflex Anoxic Seizures (STARS)

PO Box 175
Stratford upon Avon CV37 8YD
Tel: 01789 450564
E-mail: trudie@stars.org.uk
www.stars.org.uk

Synsostosis *see Microcephaly*

Systemic arthritis *see Arthritis*

Systemic lupus erythematosus

Systemic lupus erythematosus (SLE) is a rare autoimmune disease that can affect many of the body's organs in older children and teenagers. Sufferers might have a skin rash, fever, hair loss, *Anaemia*, *Arthritis*, kidney (*Glomerulonephritis*), heart (*Myocarditis*) and lung problems. The brain can also be affected and the liver and spleen might become enlarged. Treatment is with steroids and other immune suppressing agents.

Children with SLE can be educated in mainstream and special schools. The extent to which SLE affects schooling depends on the medical interventions required. School-based *Interdisciplinary working* might be necessary for some children, while community medical services will manage others. Effective links with parents and good pastoral arrangements will provide the child with physical and emotional support.

Children with SLE will need access to the same curriculum as their peers (see *Arthritis*, *Physical disability*, *Congenital heart diseases*). Special arrangements will probably be needed to provide access to physically demanding sporting activities, including a place to rest when or if tired. The safety measures for all pupils are generally sufficient.

Overall, children with SLE have a condition that from time to time can interfere with their education.

Useful links
Lupus UK
St James House
Eastern Road
Romford RM1 3NH
Tel: 01708 731251

T

Tachyarrhythmia *see* Tachycardia

Tachycardia

Tachycardia is the name given to a fast heart rate. Some children have abnormal conduction of the minute electrical impulses that normally stimulate the heart to beat in a coordinated way (tachyarrhythmia). In tachycardia there might be abnormal conduction pathways in the heart. Treatment can be with drugs or by disrupting the abnormal conduction pathways.

Children with tachycardia might have sudden, recurrent attacks at school, which might leave the child feeling faint, breathless or anxious (see *Congenital heart diseases*).

TB *see* Tuberculosis

Tetralogy of Fallot

Tetralogy of Fallot is a condition of the heart where there is the combination of a *Ventricular septal defect*, *Pulmonary stenosis* and overgrowth of the muscles of the right pumping chamber and where the main artery (aorta) lies over the hole between the pumping chambers. The condition can cause symptoms soon after birth or can cause increasing symptoms of blueness (cyanosis), breathlessness and growth problems through infancy. The treatment is operative and leads to complete resolution of the early symptoms in most cases (see *Congenital heart diseases*).

Thalassaemia

Thalassaemia is a form of anaemia caused by abnormal haemoglobin that causes the red blood cells to turn over more quickly than normal. The bone marrow and other parts of the body that manufacture the red blood cells work harder than normal, causing enlargement of the liver and spleen and enlargement of the bones of the skull and face (bossing). Children with enlarged spleen are at increased risk of damaging this abdominal organ, which is normally hidden under the rib cage; this might need to be taken into account when planning activities with physical contact or rough and tumble play/sport.

Treatment is with regular blood transfusions and infusions (slow injections of medication over a long period of time) to prevent iron overload from the repeated transfusions.

Children with thalassaemia can be educated in mainstream and special schools. School-based *Interdisciplinary working* might be necessary for some children, while community medical services will manage others. Some children will need to carry a syringe pump in which case there might be environmental factors to consider.

Thalassaemia might mean some children experience long and frequent periods of illness together with complex courses of treatment. Frequent absence from school for time-consuming treatments can lead to staff having low expectations of children's achievements and school friendships will be disrupted. It is important to explore all possible ways of supporting children who are regularly absent and to provide a range of ways to help them catch up with work; this becomes very important where children are mid-syllabus for externally accredited examinations.

Good links with parents and effective pastoral systems will support the severely affected child in all aspects of their school life. Children who are mildly affected are unlikely to need any different attention to their peers.

Useful links
Thalassaemia Support
19 The Broadway
Southgate Circus
London N14 6PH
Tel: 020 8882 0011
E-mail: OFFICE@UKTS.ORG

Threadworms *see* Worms

Tics

Tics are involuntary contractions of muscles that can worsen at times of stress or anxiety. There is a very wide range of severity so that many people with the condition might never need to seek medical attention, while others have a socially disabling condition (see *Tourette syndrome*). Many affected children have little choice in class but to make the small irresistible movements that are known as tics. Sometimes they can repress these, but it is helpful to provide a secluded spot where they can release their symptoms. Typically, tics increase as a result of tension or stress, and decrease with relaxation or when focusing on an absorbing task.

Children with tics can be educated in

mainstream and special schools. Some children will need school-based *Interdisciplinary working* while community medical services will manage others. Effective links with parents and good pastoral arrangements will provide the child with support.

Children with tics will need access to the same curriculum as their peers. The curriculum should not need to be modified for children because they have tics.

Tinnitus

Tinnitus is the word for noises that are heard in the head such as buzzing, ringing, whistling, hissing, and other sounds that do not come from an external source. Children who have tinnitus can show a number of symptoms that affect their learning. They are likely to present classroom behaviour problems, have unexplained physical responses and appear not to pay attention. It is possible for children with tinnitus to become severely depressed.

Children with tinnitus can be educated in mainstream and special schools. School-based *Interdisciplinary working* involving an educational psychologist and possibly a psychiatrist might be necessary for some children, while community medical services will manage others. Effective links with parents and good pastoral arrangements will provide support for these children.

A school should ensure that there are good pastoral support systems in place and that there is a whole-school approach to support the child with tinnitus. Work with peers might be necessary so that they understand the condition and do not overreact to situations that are beyond their immediate control. A withdrawal room can be useful as it will minimise interruptions to lessons. Some children will be affected more in specific circumstances; these might be physical, social or emotional, and it is sensible to learn about these in order to provide the best learning arrangements and to create safe and secure situations.

Useful links
The British Tinnitus Association
Ground Floor, Unit 5
Acorn Business Park
Woodseats Close
Sheffield S8 0TB
Tel: 0114 250 9933
Tel: 0845 450 0321 (Freephone Helpline)
Fax: 0114 258 7059
E-mail: bta@tinnitus.org.uk
www.tinnitus.org.uk

RNID Tinnitus Helpline
Castle Cavendish Works
Norton Street
Radford
Nottingham NG7 5PN
Tel: 0808 808 6666 (Freephone Helpline)
Tel: 0808 808 0007 (Free Textphone)
www.rnid.org.uk

Toe walking

Toe walking is sometimes seen in younger children when they first learn to walk. Usually it quickly settles but in some children it persists, causing problems with mobility and stability. This can be due to abnormal tone in the muscles or shortening of the tendon at the back of the ankle (the Achilles tendon). Physiotherapy can help, following assessment by a doctor to exclude other causes of increased tone in the muscles.

The advice and considerations about the school environment found under *Physical disability* will apply.

Useful links
STEPS
Lymm Court
11 Eagle Brow
Lymm WA13 0LP
Tel: 01925 757525
E-mail: info@steps-charity.org.uk
www.steps-charity.org.uk/

Tonsillitis

Tonsillitis is an infection affecting the tonsils. The tonsils are lumps of tissue that sit at the back of the mouth and act as a defence mechanism against the viruses and bacteria in the air. Infected tonsils swell and are associated with a sore throat and difficulty in swallowing. Treatment can be with fluids and paracetamol and also sometimes antibiotics.

This condition is usually managed by general practitioners and might include time in hospital or the interventions of community medical services. Effective links with parents and good pastoral arrangements might be needed. It is unlikely that the curriculum should be modified for children because they have tonsillitis; however, some children will be absent from school while receiving treatment.

Tourette syndrome

Tourette syndrome is a condition where tics of the muscles occur involuntarily. Children can demonstrate a range of symptoms including eye blinking, repeated throat clearing or sniffing, arm thrusting, kicking movements, shoulder shrugging or jumping. It might be accompanied by grunts, *Echolalia*, offensive gestures, and sometimes by involuntary swearing. These more often appear in the primary phase and vary from very mild to severe; the majority of cases fall into the mild category. Children with Tourette syndrome as a group have the same IQ range as the population at large, although a larger proportion have special educational needs. It is usually the case that it is linked to some other conditions, for example attention problems, impulsiveness and learning disabilities. Most children manage school well provided there is a good pastoral system and advice from relevant professionals. School-based *Interdisciplinary working* involving speech and language therapists might be necessary for some children, while community medical services will manage others. Teachers and class-based support staff will need to find ways of accommodating the irresistible elements of the condition. Many children have little choice and must make the small irresistible movements that are known as tics. Sometimes they can repress these but it is helpful to provide a secluded spot where they can release their symptoms. Typically, tics increase as a result of tension or stress and decrease with relaxation, or when focusing on an absorbing task.

Some children can have obsessions that consist of repetitive unwanted or bother-

some thoughts. They will need time and space to work through these in the ways that have proved most successful. Children can exhibit compulsions and ritualistic behaviours that occur when they feel that something must be done over and over and/or in a certain way. Examples include touching an object with one hand after touching it with the other hand to 'even things up' or repeatedly checking things, such as whether a book is in their school bag. Children sometimes beg teachers or staff to repeat a sentence many times until it 'sounds right'.

Some children might show signs of *Attention deficit disorder* before Tourette symptoms appear. Children can have difficulty with concentration; failing to finish what is started; not listening; being easily distracted; often acting before thinking; shifting constantly from one activity to another and general fidgeting. They will need a great deal of supervision and support. At times it might be useful to have strategies such as using different rooms to help a child 'settle'. Similarly children may have difficulties with impulse control that can result in rare instances of aggressive behaviours or socially inappropriate acts; children can be defiant and at times very angry.

Some children will have perceptual problems and need additional support with basic formal skills such as reading and writing and mathematics. The use of tape recorders, typewriters, or computers for reading and writing problems are useful. Special arrangements will probably be needed for some teaching and exams to take place in a different room if vocal tics are a problem.

Useful links
Tourette Syndrome (UK) Association
PO Box 26149
Dunfermline KY12 9WT
Tel: 01892 669151
E-mail: enquiries@tsa.org.uk
www.tsa.org.uk

Tracheo-oesophageal fistula

Tracheo-oesophageal fistula is a congenital condition where the baby is born with an abnormal gullet (oesophagus) and windpipe. Often the gullet does not connect to the stomach but instead to the windpipe. Sometime there is an abnormal connection between the windpipe and gullet, causing choking and feeding difficulties. Treatment is surgical and involves reconstructing the gullet and windpipe. Children might be left with residual feeding, speech and breathing difficulties, which can persist until school age. The condition can occur with other abnormalities.

Children with tracheo-oesophageal fistula can be educated in mainstream and special schools. The extent to which it affects schooling depends on the success of the repair and its consequences. School-based *Interdisciplinary working* might be necessary for some children, while community medical services will manage others. Effective links with parents and good pastoral arrangements will provide the child with support.

Some children with tracheo-oesophageal fistula will need a modified curriculum because of their learning difficulties (see *Physical disability*). Overall children with tracheo-oesophageal fistula have a condition that can effect their education.

Useful links
TOFS (Tracheo-Oesophageal Fistula Support)
St George's Centre
91 Victoria Road
Netherfield
Nottingham NG4 2NN
Tel: 0115 961 3092
E-mail: info@tofs.org.uk
www.tofs.org.uk

Transverse myelitis

Transverse myelitis is a condition where a localised part of the spinal cord is inflamed, together with the nerves that emerge from that portion of the spinal column. It can lead to permanent nerve problems posing similar difficulties with mobility, toileting and self-care as children with *Spina bifida* have. If more nerves higher up in the spine become affected during the course of the illness then the child might have a condition known as Guillain–Barré syndrome. This can cause problems with breathing as the nerves that control the respiratory muscles become affected. Most children with this rare condition recover fully in time.

Children with transverse myelitis can be educated in mainstream and special schools. School-based *Interdisciplinary working* involving the advice of a physiotherapist and an occupational therapist might be necessary for some children, while others will have their condition managed by community medical services. Effective links with parents and good pastoral arrangements will provide the child with support.

Children with transverse myelitis will need access to the same curriculum as their peers. Some children will experience periods of restricted mobility and will need exercises designed by a physiotherapist and perhaps specialised equipment as recommended by an occupational therapist. Frequent absence from school and time-consuming treatments can lead to staff having low expectations. It is important to explore all possible ways of supporting children who are regularly absent and to provide a range of ways to help them catch up with work; this becomes very important where children are mid-syllabus for externally accredited examinations. The curriculum should not need to be modified for children because they have transverse myelitis; however, some children will be absent from school while receiving treatment.

Useful links

Brain and Spine Foundation
7 Winchester House
Cranmer Road
Kennington Park
London SW9 6EJ
Tel: 020 7793 5900
www.brainandspine.org.uk

Transverse Myelitis Association
www.myelitis.org/local/uk/Introduction.htm

Treacher Collins syndrome

Treacher Collins syndrome is a genetic condition that affects the appearance of the face owing to underdevelopment of part of the facial structures and organs. Children might have drooping eyelids (a condition known as ptosis), microtia or *Anotia*, and occasional problems such as *Cleft lip and palate*.

Children with Treacher Collins syndrome can be educated in mainstream and special schools and could have had some or all corrective surgery completed preschool (see *Disfigurement and difference*). Periodic surgical treatment to ears and eyes can cause fluctuations in sensory acuity. Residual problems can result in difficulty with speech in which case working with a speech and language therapist is very important. School-based *Interdisciplinary working* might be necessary for some children, while community medical services will manage others. Effective links with parents and good pastoral arrangements will provide support for these children (see *Speech and language problems, Crouzon's syndrome, Conductive hearing loss* and *Cleft lip and palate.*

Prolonged admissions to hospital are likely and close liaison with hospital schools and/or outreach services can help provide continuity of the curriculum. A school needs good systems of support and opportunities for children to catch up after periods of absence. Children needing frequent absence from school and time-consuming treatments can lead to staff having low expectations of them and school friendships will be disrupted. It is important to explore all possible ways of supporting children who are absent for long periods and to provide a range of ways to help them catch up with work; this becomes very important where children are mid-syllabus for externally accredited examinations.

Tricuspid atresia

Tricuspid atresia is a congenital heart defect where the blood is prevented from being pumped into the lungs by the right side of the heart because of a missing connection between the collecting and pumping chambers. The right ventricle (pumping chamber) is also often underdeveloped. This causes the baby to be blue (cyanosed). Early treatment involves an operation to allow more blood to pump through the lungs. Later treatment involves a series of operations to enable blood returning from the body to flow directly through the lungs (without the heart having to pump it through) and to let the left ventricle pump the oxygenated blood around the body (the Fontan procedure). Children with these problems might find it hard to take part in physical exercise (see *Congenital heart diseases*).

Tuberculosis

Tuberculosis (TB) is an infection that affects mainly the lungs, but can affect other organs of the body. The lung infection can produce cough, temperatures, night sweating and weight loss. In younger children it can hamper growth. People with untreated infections of the lung (pulmonary TB) can infect others. Infection is usually spread when contact has been close or prolonged. There are occasional outbreaks at schools. Treatment in the UK is very successful with a combination of antibiotics that have to be taken for several months continuously. Vaccination against TB is part of the UK immunisation schedule. In some cases, TB can affect the gut, bones, urinary tract and the nervous system.

Children with tuberculosis can be educated in mainstream and special schools. The extent to which tuberculosis infection affects schooling depends on the severity of the condition and on any medical interventions required. This condition is usually managed by community medical services. Effective links with parents and good pastoral arrangements might be needed.

It is unlikely that the curriculum should be modified for children because they have TB; however, some children will be absent from school while receiving treatment.

Tuberous sclerosis

Tuberous sclerosis is caused by an abnormal gene that results in the child having multiple growths of tissue in the brain, eye, skin and kidney. The heart can also be affected. In many children it results in *Epilepsy* and learning difficulties. There are also marks on the skin and a red rash develops over the face. The facial rash can be treated with laser therapy.

Children with tuberous sclerosis can be educated in mainstream and special schools. The extent to which tuberous sclerosis affects schooling depends on how children are affected. School-based *Interdisciplinary working* including the advice of speech and language therapists and/or specialist language teachers in designing and carrying out a communication programme might be required. Effective links with parents and good pastoral arrangements will provide the child with support.

Some children with tuberous sclerosis will need a highly specialised provision with suitable environments and trained staff because of their learning difficulties (see *Epilepsy*). Some children will have specific language difficulties with a significant number of children having no speech. Some children will be overactive, have a limited attention span and show inflexibility. Generally the curriculum should be significantly modified for children because they have tuberous sclerosis.

Useful links
Tuberous Sclerosis Association
Little Barnsley Farm
Catshill
Bromsgrove B61 0NQ
Tel: 01527 871898
E-mail: secretary@tuberous-sclerosis.org
www.tuberous-sclerosis.org

Chat area for people living with tuberous sclerosis:
reecemart2001/my homepage

Turner syndrome

Turner syndrome occurs when a girl is born with just one X chromosome (females normally have two). This leads to some babies having heart defects such as *Coarctation of the aorta*. Others have kidney problems. Children are short and do not enter puberty normally as the ovaries are underdeveloped.

Girls with Turner syndrome will usually have their educational needs met in a mainstream school. The school's pastoral arrangements should be excellent particularly as their classmates move through puberty. When this is happening, schools will need to liaise carefully with the family and possibly seek the advice and support of trained counsellors.

Girls with Turner syndrome are normal intellectually but might have particular problems visualising objects in relation to each other because of visual memory and visual–motor coordination. This difficulty might show up in poor performance in mathematics, geometry, and tasks requiring manual dexterity or sense of direction. It might be sensible for girls to be assessed by an educational psychologist so that necessary adjustments can be built into their programmes.

The language skills of girls with Turner syndrome are generally good. They are likely to read well and can be good contributors in classroom discussions. The condition might not have any impact on the learning of some girls, although others can have poor social skills, low self-esteem and can become socially withdrawn.

It is unlikely that the curriculum should be significantly modified due to the condition.

Useful links
SOFT UK
48 Froggatts Ride
Walmley
Sutton Coldfield B76 2TQ

Tel: 0121 351 3122
E-mail: enquiries@soft.org.uk
www.soft.org.uk

The Turners Syndrome Support Society (UK)
1/8 Irving Court
Hardgate
Clydebank G81 6BA
Tel: 01389 380385/872511
E-mail: Turner.Syndrome@tss.org.uk
www. tss.org.uk

U

Ulcerative colitis

Ulcerative colitis is a chronic inflammatory disease of the lower part of the bowel (rectum and colon). This produces bleeding, loose stools with mucus, and discomfort. Children might not grow adequately and diarrhoea can interfere with normal school activities. It is an illness punctuated by periods of remission from the disease and then exacerbations. Some children also have *Arthritis* and rashes associated with the condition. Treatment includes drugs by mouth, and surgery is sometimes required in more severe cases.

Children with ulcerative colitis can be educated in mainstream and special schools. School-based *Interdisciplinary working* might be necessary for some children, while community medical services will manage others. Effective links with parents and good pastoral arrangements will provide the child with support.

Some children with ulcerative colitis need special arrangements to get to toilets when they need to and need to rest in a room that is quiet at break and lunch times. It is unlikely that the curriculum should be modified for children because they have ulcerative colitis.

Useful links
National Association for Colitis and Crohn's Disease
PO Box 205
St Albans AL1 1AB
www.digestivedisorders.org.uk/leaflets/coli tis.html

Undescended testes

Testicles that fail to migrate from the abdomen where they first develop down into the scrotum are called undescended testes. The testes need to be in the scrotum to ensure normal fertility. Surgery is used to bring the testicle down and attach it within the scrotum.

Boys with undescended testes can be educated in mainstream and special schools. Most boys will have their condition straightforwardly corrected by medical services. Effective links with parents and good pastoral arrangements will provide the child with support. It is unlikely that the curriculum should be modified because boys have undescended testes.

Upper respiratory tract infection

Upper respiratory tract infection is the term applied to viral and bacterial infections affecting the ears, nose, tonsils, throat and larynx, for example colds, sore throats, ear and chest infections. These are extremely common in children and are at their peak during the winter months. Treatment of viral upper respiratory tract infections is usually with fluids, paracetamol or ibuprofen. The conditions usually get better in time on their own.

General practitioners usually treat these conditions. Effective links with parents and good pastoral arrangements might be needed. It is unlikely that the curriculum should be modified for children because they have upper respiratory tract infections.

Urinary tract infections

Urinary tract infections occur when bacteria grow in the normally sterile urine. The infection can affect the kidneys (pyelonephritis) or bladder (cystitis). Both sexes can be affected. The infection can cause the child to have a fever, feel unwell and vomit, and there might be abdominal or loin pain. There is usually pain on passing urine (dysuria) and the urine often smells offensive and might be cloudy or blood-stained. Treatment is with antibiotics and fluids. Once a child has had a urinary tract infection, investigations will probably be performed to ensure that the kidneys and bladder are normal. Some children might need *Prophylactic antibiotics* following the infection while investigations are carried out. Children with, or recovering from, a urinary tract infection might face temporary continence difficulties.

Children with urinary tract infection can be educated in mainstream and special schools. Most children will have their condition managed by community medical services. Effective links with parents and good pastoral arrangements will provide the child with support. It is unlikely that the curriculum should be modified for children because they have a urinary tract infection.

Useful links
National Kidney Federation
6 Stanley Street
Worksop S81 7HX
Tel: 0845 601 0209
E-mail: helpline@kidney.org.uk
www.kidney.org.uk

Nephronline
E-mail: info@nephronline.org
www.nephronline.org/

Usher syndrome

Usher syndrome is a rare syndrome causing both hearing and visual impairment. There are different types affecting children at different ages, and this can result in some children never learning to speak because of hearing impairment present from birth. The visual difficulties are caused by *Retinitis pigmentosa* and occur later on in childhood (see *Deafblind*).

Children with Usher syndrome will have their educational needs met in schools where they can be taught by highly specialised staff in an environment that supports their learning. School-based *Interdisciplinary working* including specialist teachers and a specialist educational psychologist will be necessary. Effective links with parents and good pastoral arrangements will be needed to provide the child with support. Deafblind children need highly specialised support at the earliest possible age. Extreme isolation can lead to difficulties in communication and therefore in the development of learning skills. Developing communication skills is very important, requiring intensive individual work. Children can be taught a range of communication systems including objects of reference, symbols, sign language and Braille. Many children will need an intervenor in order to access the world and to learn. A trained intervenor will motivate the child and become their eyes and ears providing feedback from the world. This complex role is necessary for deafblind children and requires high levels of skill and dedication.

Useful links
www.deafblind.com/index.html#bsl
A Deafblindness Web Resource site owned and maintained by James Gallagher.

www.qca.org.uk/onq/schools/inclusion_wawn.asp
Shared World Different Experiences: Designing the

Curriculum for Pupils who are Deafblind (QCA/99/420) £6.

Usher Resources
Sense
11–13 Clifton Terrace
London N4 3SR
Tel: 020 7272 7774
E-mail: enquiries@sense.org.uk
www.sense.org.uk

V

Vasculitis *see* Arteritis

Ventricular septal defect

Ventricular septal defect (VSD) is a hole between the pumping chambers of the heart. It can cause breathlessness, particularly on exercise, and in younger children can affect growth. Long-term or severe defects can damage the lungs and make repair of the heart impossible (see *Eisenmenger syndrome*). The flow of blood through the hole can increase the risk of infections in the heart (endocarditis). Some holes close of their own accord. Others require surgical closure, which is curative. This condition can coexist with other heart defects.

For the child at school, the main impact of a large defect will be on their ability to take part in strenuous physical exercise (see *Congenital heart diseases*).

Ventriculoperitoneal shunt

This is a device that consists of a series of tubes and valves. It is inserted into the fluid systems of the brain (the ventricles) and allows cerebrospinal fluid to drain from the brain into the abdominal cavity via the device. The fluid is then absorbed by the body. It is used to control raised intracranial pressure that can occur with *Spina bifida*, *Hydrocephalus* or *Brain tumours*. The shunts can become infected but usually the underlying condition itself for which the shunt has been inserted is more of an issue.

Children with a ventriculoperitoneal shunt can be educated in mainstream and special schools. The extent to which this condition affects schooling depends on the medical interventions and monitoring required. Some children will need frequent and regular visits to hospital and will need exercises designed by a physiotherapist. School-based *Interdisciplinary working* involving a physiotherapist and an occupational therapist might be necessary for some children, while community medical services will manage others. Effective links with parents and good pastoral arrangements will provide the child with support.

Children with a ventriculoperitoneal shunt will need access to the same curriculum as their peers (see *Spina bifida*, *Hydrocephalus* and *Physical disability*). Frequent absence from school and time-consuming treatments can lead to low expectations. It is important to explore all possible ways of supporting children who are regularly absent and to provide a range of ways to help them catch up with work. This becomes very important where children are mid-syllabus for externally accredited examinations. Some children will spend long periods in wheelchairs; therefore access to classrooms and other school buildings needs to be good.

Useful links
Association for Spina Bifida and Hydrocephalus
42 Park Road
Peterborough PE1 2UQ
Tel: 01733 555988
E-mail: postmaster@asbah.org
www.asbah.org/

Verbal dyspraxia

Children with verbal dyspraxia have problems ordering the components of speech
and they struggle with the 'motor plan' for
correctly pronouncing and saying words. So
children might know what they want to say,
but cannot say it (see *Speech disorder* and
Dyspraxia). School-based *Interdisciplinary
working* including the advice of a speech and
language therapist might be necessary for
some children. Effective links with parents
and good pastoral arrangements will provide
the child with support.

Children with verbal dyspraxia have a
limited speech sound repertoire and they
tend to use a simple syllable such as 'la' or
'ma' to stand for almost everything. They
might use short single words well, but as
soon as two or three words in a row are used
they drop all the ending sounds of the
words. Young children unable to think of
words to use to enter into play with friends
might evolve inappropriate social strategies,
such as hitting or disrupting play. In older
children, difficulty finding the right words
might show up as shyness or a tendency to
rely on 'I don't know' as a response to questions. Problems with the retrieval,
coordination and articulation of words all
make communication very difficult and
therefore a barrier to learning. Most children
who receive high quality intervention will
eventually be competent oral communica-
tors. In severe cases, *Alternative and
augmentative communication* (AAC) will be
needed.

It is vital to give a child confidence and
support, so teachers and class-based staff
will need to accept whatever the child says

and, if it is right, give praise. Try to make the
child feel as good as possible about their
speech and self-esteem. Give positive reinforcement to the child's attempts at
communication and accuracy. Where possible provide a correct model so that the
message can be stated correctly. Support the
child in the programme provided by the
speech and language therapist where possible, and integrate this into lessons.
Sometimes the speech and language therapist will advise on the use of a system of
assisted communication such as signing, use
of symbols or a speech output device, as
these are particularly valuable where a child
has good comprehension but poor expression.

Overall children with verbal dyspraxia
have a condition that will to some extent
affect their education.

Useful links
Afasic
2nd Floor
50–52 Great Sutton Street
London EC1V 0DJ
Tel: 020 7490 9410
E-mail: info@afasic.org.uk
www.afasic.org.uk

Vernal conjunctivitis *see* Conjunctivitis

Vertigo

Vertigo is the feeling of things spinning
around. It is often associated with unsteadiness, nausea and sometimes vomiting. Some
children have vertigo associated with ear

infections and conditions such as *Labyrinthitis* and glue ear *(see Otitis media)*. Others get sudden attacks of vertigo without any apparent reason (benign paroxysmal vertigo). Occasionally older children will get vertigo as part of *Migraine*. Vertigo can affect motor skills and confidence.

Children with vertigo can be educated in mainstream and special schools. School-based *Interdisciplinary working* might be necessary for some children, while community medical services will manage others. Effective links with parents and good pastoral arrangements will provide support for these children.

Vesicoureteric reflux

Vesicoureteric reflux or reflux nephropathy is a condition when damage to the developing kidneys (usually in the first two years of life) is caused by urine flowing back up towards the kidneys from the bladder. There is an increased risk of infection of the urine and the infections are more likely to scar the kidneys and potentially can reduce their ability to function normally. Children usually grow out of this tendency. Children might receive antibiotics to prevent infections from taking hold (*Prophylactic antibiotics*); some severe cases might require surgery to prevent the back flow of urine. For the child this can mean time off school and occasional incontinence.

Children with vesicoureteric reflux can be educated in mainstream and special schools. School-based *Interdisciplinary working* might be necessary for some children, although most will have their condition managed by medical services and it will not adversely affect schooling. Effective links with parents and good pastoral arrangements will provide the child with support. It is unlikely that the curriculum should be modified for children because they have vesicoureteric reflux; however, some children will be absent from school while receiving treatment.

Useful links
National Kidney Federation
6 Stanley Street
Worksop S81 7HX
Tel: 0845 601 0209
E-mail: helpline@kidney.org.uk
www.kidney.org.uk

Nephronline
E-mail: info@nephronline.org
www.nephronline.org/

Visual impairment

Arrangements for meeting the needs of pupils with a visual impairment will generally include advice from a range of professionals looking at every aspect of the child's life (see *Interdisciplinary working*). Advice from assessment is the first place to start when thinking about the educational programme. It is sensible to look at the child, the environment and the curriculum.

Children with low vision have substantial visual impairment but nevertheless are able to use a significant amount of their remaining visual function. Many different conditions that affect either the eyes locally or other parts of the nervous system can cause this difficulty (see under individual entries for *Achromatopsia, Albinism, Cataract, Coloboma, Cortical blindness, Glaucoma, Nystagmus, Optic atrophy, Refractive error, Retinoblastoma, Retinitis pigmentosa* and *Retinopathy of prematurity*). Problems with vision can affect development of movement, coordination and speech.

Consideration should be given to the implications of visual impairment on physical, cognitive, emotional, and social and language development and their effect upon the child's independence. Appropriate strategies should be implemented to enhance functional vision. It is important to develop secondary senses (hearing, touch, etc.) when a primary sense is impaired. Working closely with a pupil should identify the best point of vision. It is very important that pupils use their preferred way of seeing and can explain the importance of this to others. The monitoring of a pupil's well-being during the school day is vital, as fatigue and anxiety can affect vision; for example where reading is slow more time is needed for work to be completed.

Mobility arrangements will be individually determined through the advice from a mobility officer/specialist and/or the advice of a specialist teacher of the visually impaired. It is almost certain that an ongoing mobility programme will need maintaining and extending. Careful planning is needed to prepare children for changes or new environments, for example at times of transition or school trips. Hooples, canes and sticks are made for all kinds of needs including lightweight and foldaway versions. Guide dogs are not usually available until people are at least 16 years old.

Attention should be given to the school environment as a whole, including the classrooms, teaching areas used and the media used for presenting the curriculum. The colour codes for school paintwork can be made compatible with the needs of visually impaired users. For example:

- Use the same colours for common areas with architrave and doorframes picked out in contrasting colours.
- Classroom doors and toilets can be colour-coded.
- Corridors could have guiding strips attached to walls.
- Perspectives might be difficult to judge so care must be taken with stairs, uneven areas or places with different levels.
- Similar attention can be paid to the décor of classrooms with a view to assisting/augmenting any vision that a student might have.
- Routes or aisles between desks can be marked out with coloured plastic tape.
- Good lighting with reduced glare is important.
- A white ceiling and light coloured walls will make the best use of any available light.
- Notice boards need to be at eye level and can be provided in a single contrasting colour.
- Use a white, black or colour board and take care with the colour of pen, felt or marker to be used.

Simple things such as how a child will know the time should be considered. It can be difficult for some children to safely manage drinks and other liquids. There are some good liquid sensors available from the Royal

National Institute for the Blind that assist with this process. Specific visual aids might be required for some children. If the pupil uses low vision aids (LVAs), then these need to be stored somewhere that is easily accessible. To make the most of a low vision aid they will need supported opportunities for regular practice; this might have an implication for the school timetable. It is important to keep spectacles and other lenses clean. An optician will give helpful advice. It is very important to get the right cleaners; detergents and incorrect cleaners can damage expensive plastic lenses. For reading, children could use stand magnifiers, hand-held magnifiers or special reading glasses, such as bifocals with a strong reading lens or telescopic reading lenses clipped over glasses. Some children use monoculars (small hand-held telescopes). Older students might use bioptic lens systems, which can improve reading and distance vision.

It is usually necessary to design and produce materials in the appropriate medium for pupils with visual impairment, for example objects of reference, tactile formations, Braille and large print using available media. Sensory materials need to be carefully considered and introduced systematically within a regime where there is regular opportunity for reinforcement and consolidation.

To maximise the learning opportunities of this group of children, media, materials and resources can be presented from the preferred point of view for the pupil. Sometimes it is useful for the pupil to sit at a particular angle to the board or source of presentation. Materials are better enlarged and appropriately contrasted: it is more sensible to allow the pupil their own materials rather than expect them to share. Larger monitors/screens should be considered – children who wish to read a lot and those who require large magnification or greater contrast between print and paper might benefit from a closed circuit television (CCTV) magnifier. When using CCTV, try white letters on black background to reduce glare.

For reading and finding things out, large print books should be made available or borrowed. Print can be magnified using low vision aids or by making enlargements on a photocopier. Where colour vision is intact, contrast is probably more important than size of print. Some children will find it helpful to use a ruler to mark the line or to place a piece of black card with a slit in it revealing the line of print. For some children access to a sensory room that can be darkened is invaluable. In this setting presentations can be specially lit and children can practise and develop tracking and scanning skills.

To support curriculum access, information using recorded media will be required. There is a wide range of recorded material for the cassette and compact disc player. Cassette and compact disc players are widely available in schools – it is very important to encourage the use of recorded media, as this will provide a lifetime access to information. A vast range of Talking Books, Magazines and Newspapers is available for purchase or loan from local groups and outlets.

Reading text by touch is a useful skill requiring specialised teaching. The two systems most often used are Braille and Moon. Braille letters are formed with different combinations of six dots; Moon letters are based on the shapes of conventionally printed letters and therefore ideal for those who already have knowledge of print.

Writing is aided by attention to size and contrast; there are many helpful aids available, such as exercise books and paper with bold lines, or writing frames to help with position and alignment. Writing needs to be large, bold, well spaced and produced, for example, with felt tip or marker pens. The use of word processors and computers provide flexible access to a means of providing the written word, and teaching keyboard skills is helped through a large number of adapted keyboards. The rapid development of voice-activated software will provide additional means of producing text. When using computers it is sensible to attend carefully to the configuration of colours, contrast, size and shape of fonts.

Advice can be sought on applications of microtechnology in meeting the needs of children and young people with visual impairment. There is no doubt that the advances in every aspect of microtechnology will provide increased access and opportunity for children with little or no sight.

Standardised assessment tests (SATs) might need to be photocopied and enlarged. There are three types of modified paper normally available – Braille, enlarged and modified large print. There is useful advice on this on the Royal National Institute for the Blind's website (see below).

Careful consideration of PE and sporting activities is required. For example, some pupils are better at throwing balls than catching them. Large and small apparatus need to be of contrasting colour or perhaps with leading edges highlighted. Highly polished hall floors can reflect unwelcome glare. Swimming, aerobics, gymnastics, track events, horse riding and skiing are examples of sports that can be enjoyed with minimal adaptations.

Other interagency arrangements and linkages are important. Many children are registered as blind or partially sighted. A specialist social worker, rehabilitation (mobility) officer, or low vision therapist, might be involved at different stages during the child's school career. Ongoing involvement of a peripatetic teacher of the visually impaired and input from ophthalmology professionals is desirable to design an effective educational programme – see *Interdisciplinary working*.

It can be very helpful for the affected child to work with sighted peers, encouraging them to be aware of the implications of the partial sight of their classmate. Sighted peers can greatly assist with encouragement and support. Take care over arrangements such as these, as independence and confidence are important.

Useful links
Hands and Eyes
A USA specialist teacher maintains this useful online newsletter for teachers and caregivers of visually impaired students and their friends. It includes art, cooking and manipulative activities that visually impaired students can do individually or in small groups. It is for teachers and support staff in need of ideas for classroom activities and is particularly useful for pupils with multiple impairments such as developmental disability and motor impairment.
www.home.earthlink.net/~vharris/

RNIB Education Information Services
224 Great Portland Street
London W1N 6AA
Tel: 020 7388 1266
E-mail: webmaster@rnib.org.uk
www.rnib.org.uk
*RNIB's curriculum information service offers infor-
mation and advice to all professionals supporting a
visually impaired child in mainstream or special
schools.*
www.rnib.org.uk/curriculum/

http://rnib.org.uk/curriculum/exams.htm
*RNIB's accessing technology pages provide informa-
tion about applications of technology in employment,
at study and in leisure.*
www.rnib.org.uk/technology/

V.I. Guide
*This site contains information on many topics relat-
ing to parenting and teaching a child with visual
impairments.*
www.viguide.com/

W

Wheeze

Wheeze is heard as air is forced out of the lungs through narrowed breathing tubes. It is often described as sounding like air coming from bellows and is most commonly seen in children suffering from *Asthma*. It is very common and can, if untreated, lead to very severe breathlessness and distress. Treatment is mainly with inhalers that dilate the narrowed airways and/or prevent the airways narrowing in the first place.

Children who wheeze can be educated in mainstream and special schools. These conditions are usually simply managed by community medical services. Effective links with parents and good pastoral arrangements might be needed.

Children who wheeze should not need different curriculum arrangements to their peers. Staff should be aware of the supportive things they can do where there are allergies. Some families will want to explore diets excluding certain foods; schools can help parents by managing access to permitted foods and supervising snacks at break times and by observing children over time.

Useful links
Action against Allergy
PO Box 278
Twickenham TW1 4QQ
Tel: 020 8892 2711
E-mail:
AAA@actionagainstallergy.freeserve.co.uk
www.actionagainstallergy.co.uk

Breathe Easy
British Lung Foundation
78 Hatton Garden
London EC1N 8LD
Tel: 020 7831 5831
E-mail: blf@britishlungfoundation.com
www.lunguk.org

British Allergy Foundation
Deepdene House
30 Bellegrove Road
Welling DA16 3PY
Tel: 020 8303 8583
E-mail: info@allergyfoundation.com
www.allergyfoundation.com

National Society for Research into Allergies
and Environmental Diseases
PO Box 45
Hinckley LE10 1JY
Tel/Fax: 01455 250715
E-mail: nsra.allergy@virgin.net

Williams syndrome

Williams syndrome causes moderate to severe learning difficulties. Children might have narrowing of the main arteries from the heart to the body or the lungs. Children have a characteristic-looking face (often described as 'elfin-like') and can have difficulties with feeding and gaining weight when very young. Children have inattentiveness, motor restlessness and are sensitive to loud noises.

Children with Williams syndrome can be educated in mainstream and special schools. School-based *Interdisciplinary working* might be necessary for some children. Good pastoral arrangements should be in place to support the child. It is important to have effective liaison and communication with parents and carers.

Children can have misleadingly well developed language in contrast to their perceptual abilities and motor skills. It can be easy for staff to think that children are learning well alongside peers, but assessment might show they might need support in areas such as reading, writing, listening and mathematics. Care and attention should be given to PE and the more demanding sporting activities. Some children might have behavioural difficulties that include hyperactivity, poor concentration and attention-seeking behaviours. Poor motor skills, difficulty visualising objects in relation to each other, problems with visual memory and visual–motor coordination will mean children need differentiation particularly in practical classroom activities.

Care should be taken as some children can have poor relationships with peers yet be overfriendly with strangers. Loud unpredictable noises and persistent sounds can be problematic and so it might be necessary to look carefully at the classroom and other parts of the school and not put children near heaters or similar sources of noise. Children with Williams syndrome have a condition that will affect their educational provision.

Useful links
Williams Syndrome Foundation
161 High Street
Tonbridge TN9 1BX
Tel: 01732 365152
E-mail:
John.nelson-wsfoundation@btInternet.com
www.williams-syndrome.org.uk

Wilms tumour

Wilms tumour is a cancer of the kidney that affects young children. They may complain of a lump in the tummy or have blood in the urine. Treatment is with a combination of surgery and chemotherapy, and has a reasonably high success rate.

Children with Wilms tumour can be educated in mainstream and special schools. Generally children will be receiving treatment during their early school years. School-based *Interdisciplinary working* might be necessary for some children, while others will have their condition managed by medical services. Effective links with parents and good pastoral arrangements will provide support for these children.

Wilms tumour might mean some children experience long or frequent periods of illness together with complex courses of treatment. Frequent absence from school and time-consuming treatments can lead to staff having low expectations and disruption to friendships. It is important to explore all possible ways of supporting children who are regularly absent and to provide a range of ways to help them catch up with work; this becomes very important where children are mid-syllabus for externally accredited examinations.

Side effects of treatment might need sensitive management. Children with Wilms tumour will need the same access to the curriculum as their peers, although at times they can present as underachievers because of absence from school.

Useful links
CancerBACUP

3 Bath Place
Rivington Street
London EC2A 3JR
Tel: 020 7696 9003
E-mail: info@cancerbacup.org
www.cancerbacup.org.uk

Cancer Care Society
11 The Cornmarket
Romsey SO51 8GB
Tel: 01794 830300
E-mail: info@cancercaresoc.org
www.cancercaresoc.org

Cancerlink
Macmillan Cancer Relief
89 Albert Embankment
London SE1 7UQ
Tel: 0808 808 0000
Tel: 020 7840 7840
E-mail: cancerlink@cancerlink.org.uk
www.cancerlink.org

Worms

Threadworms or pinworms (Latin name *Enterobius vermicularis*) are parasites that can infest small children. They reproduce in the gut and lay eggs around the anus, which can cause intense itching and discomfort (pruri-tis ani). When children scratch their bottoms to relieve the itching, eggs are transferred under the fingernails and can then infest other children or re-infect the child itself. The condition is easily treated, and attention to hand washing and appropriate self-care can prevent recurrence.

Children with worms can be educated in mainstream and special schools. Primary children are more likely to need support and guidance. A school-based health education programme provided by colleagues from community medical teams is helpful. Effective links with parents and good pastoral arrangements will provide the child with support.

Some young children with worms will need special arrangements in toilets and at break and lunch times. It is unlikely that the curriculum should be modified for children because they have worms.

Useful links
Community Hygiene Concern
Manor Gardens Centre
6–9 Manor Gardens
London N7 6LA
Tel: 020 7686 4321
E-mail: bugbusters2k@yahoo.co.uk
www.chc.org

Z

Zellweger syndrome

Zellweger syndrome is a rare condition causing damage to the brain and nervous system because of problems with the child's cells; parts within the cell are unable to maintain it in a healthy state. Children with this condition have movement problems (*Hypotonia*), severe learning difficulties and visual impairment. This syndrome is known as a peroxisomal disorder.

Some children with Zellweger syndrome might have their educational needs met in mainstream schools, while others will need very special care and the highly differentiated education usually found in a special school. School-based *Interdisciplinary working* involving therapists will become necessary. Effective pastoral arrangements will be needed, including giving the children and their family high levels of support and access to counselling.

The curriculum will need highly specialised input from experienced and trained specialist teachers (see *Physical disability*, *Visual impairment*, *Hearing impairment*). The educational programme will need to include access to the same curriculum as all children. Overall children with Zellweger syndrome have a condition that will significantly affect their education

Useful links
Climb
The Quadrangle
Crewe Hall
Weston Road
Crewe CW2 6UR
Tel: 0870 770 0326
E-mail: info@climb.org.uk
www.climb.org.uk

Further reading

Booth T. *et al. Index for Inclusion: Developing Learning and Participation in Schools.* Centre for Studies on Inclusive Education (CSIE), 2000.
The index is a set of materials to support schools in a process of inclusive school development.

Byers R., Rose R. *Planning the Curriculum for Pupils with Special Educational Needs.* London: David Fulton, 1996.

Coupe O'Kane, J., Goldbart, J. *Communication before Speech: Development and Assessment,* 2nd edn, London: David Fulton, 1998.

DoE Circular 9/94 DoH LAC (94) 9. *The Education of Children with Emotional and Behavioural Difficulties.*
Download address:
www.doh.gov.uk/pub/docs/lacs/93_95/9alac.pdf

DfEE Circular 14/96. *Supporting Pupils with Medical Needs in School.*
The circular sets out the legal framework and is available via the DfES website at www.dfee.gov.uk/circulars/14_96/summary.htm

DfEE Circular 10/99. *Social Inclusion: Pupil Support.*
Explains the law and good practice on pupil behaviour and discipline, reducing the risk of disaffection, school attendance and registration, detention, proper use of exclusion, and re-integration of excluded pupils

DfEE Circular 11/99. *Social Inclusion: the LEA role in Pupil Support.*
This guidance explains the administrative and legal responsibilities of LEAs for managing attendance, including legal action for enforcing attendance, for providing education outside school, for pupils at risk of exclusion, for educating and re-integrating excluded pupils and for pupil referral units.

DfES 0068/2001. *Good practice guidance, home to school transport for children with special educational needs.*

DfES 0121/2001. *Promoting Children's Mental Health within Early Years and School Settings.*
This includes examples of good practice to help school staff, working alongside mental health professionals, in early identification and intervention for pupils experiencing mental health problems. It recognises schools, often working in partnership with other agencies, can help promote the mental health of all children, and particularly those children most at risk of developing mental health problems.

DfEE/Department of Health 1996. *Supporting Pupils with Medical Needs: a Good Practice Guide.*
Written to help schools draw up policies on managing medication in schools, and to put in place effective management systems to support individual pupils with medical needs. It also contains proforma, which can be used by schools.
Download address:
www.dfes.gov.uk/medical

DfES 2001. *Access to Education for Children and Young People with Medical Needs.*
This sets out minimum national standards for the education of children who are unable to attend school because of illness or injury.
Download address:
www.dfes.gov.uk/sen/viewDocument.cf

m?dID=257

DfEE/Department of Health Joint Guidance 2000. *Guidance on the Education of Children and Young People in Public Care.*

DfES 0629/2001. *Guidance on the Education of School Age Parents.*

DfES 2001. *Inclusive Schooling – Children with Special Educational Needs.*
The document provides practical guidance on the new statutory framework for inclusion.
Download address:
www.dfes.gov.uk/sen/viewDocument.cf
m?dID=237

DfES 2001. *The SEN Code of Practice.*
Provides practical advice to Local Education Authorities, maintained schools, early education settings and others on carrying out their statutory duties to identify, assess and make provision for children's special educational needs.
Download address:
www.dfes.gov.uk/sen/index.cfm

DfES 2001. *Special Educational Needs and Disability Act 2001*
The Special Educational Needs and Disability Act 2001 *amended the* Disability Discrimination Act 1995 *so that it covers every aspect of education. The duties that apply to those who provide school education make it unlawful to discriminate, without justification, against disabled pupils and prospective pupils, in all aspects of school life.*
Download address:
www.hmso.gov.uk/acts/acts2001/20010
010.htm

DfES/QCA 1998. *Supporting the target setting process.*
This advice is intended to support schools in the setting of effective targets for pupils with special educational needs. It builds on earlier guidance published as a result of the National Foundation for Educational Research commission to develop performance criteria, in consultation with a large number of special and mainstream schools, for attainment below National Curriculum Level 3 in English and Mathematics.

Farrell, P., Balshaw, M., Polat, F. *The Management Role and Training of Learning Support Assistants.* Research Report RR161. London: DfES, 1999.

Lacey, P. 'Multidisciplinary work', in Tilstone C., Florian, L., Rose, R. (eds) *Promoting Inclusive Practice.* London: Routledge, 1998.

Lawson, H. *Practical Record Keeping,* 2nd edn. London: David Fulton, 1998.

Marvin, C. 'Individual and whole class teaching', in Tilstone, C., Florian, L., Rose, R. (eds) *Promoting Inclusive Practice.* London: Routledge, 1998.

Nind, M., Hewett, D. *Access to Communication.* London: David Fulton, 1999.

Pagliano, P. *Using a Multisensory Environment: A Practical Guide for Teachers.* London: David Fulton, 2001.

Rose, R. 'A jigsaw approach to group work'. *British Journal of Special Education* 1991, **18**(20): 54–7.

School Curriculum and Assessment Authority [now QCA]. *Planning the Curriculum for Pupils with Profound and Multiple Learning Difficulties.* London: SCAA, 1996.

Tilstone, C., Lacey, P., Porter, J., Robertson C. *Pupils with Learning Difficulties in Mainstream Schools.* London: David Fulton, 2000.

Ware, J. *Creating a Responsive Environment.* London: David Fulton, 1996.